The Social Prescribing Link Worker Model

Insights and Perspectives from Practice

Christiana Melam MBE

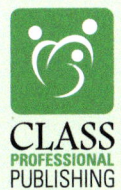

CLASS
PROFESSIONAL
PUBLISHING

Class Professional Publishing have made every effort to ensure that the information, tables, drawings and diagrams contained in this book are accurate at the time of publication. The book cannot always contain all the information necessary for determining appropriate care and cannot address all individual situations; therefore, individuals using the book must ensure they have the appropriate knowledge and skills to enable suitable interpretation. Class Professional Publishing does not guarantee, and accepts no legal liability of whatever nature arising from or connected to, the accuracy, reliability, currency or completeness of the content of The Social Prescribing Link Worker Model. Users must always be aware that such innovations or alterations after the date of publication may not be incorporated in the content. Please note, however, that Class Professional Publishing assumes no responsibility whatsoever for the content of external resources in the text or accompanying online materials.

The Social Prescribing Link Worker Model © National Association of Link Workers, 2024.

All rights reserved. Without limiting the rights under copyright reserved above, no part of this publication may be reproduced, stored in or introduced into a retrieval system, or transmitted, in any form or by any means (electronic, mechanical, photocopying, recording or otherwise) without the prior written permission of the publisher of this book.

The information presented in this book is accurate and current to the best of the authors' knowledge.

The authors and publisher, however, make no guarantee as to, and assume no responsibility for, the correctness, sufficiency or completeness of such information or recommendation.

Printing history

This first edition published in 2024.

The authors and publisher welcome feedback from the users of this book. Please contact the publisher:

Class Professional Publishing,
The Exchange, Express Park, Bristol Road, Bridgwater TA6 4RR

Telephone: 01278 472 800
Email: info@class.co.uk
Website: www.classprofessional.co.uk

Class Professional Publishing is an imprint of Class Publishing Ltd
A CIP catalogue record for this book is available from the British Library

Paperback ISBN: 9781801610001
eBook ISBN: 9781801610018
Designed and typeset by PHi Business Solutions
Printed in the UK by Hobbs

MIX
Paper from responsible sources
FSC
www.fsc.org   FSC® C020438

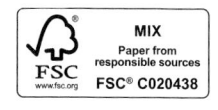

This book is printed on paper from responsible sources. Refer to local recycling guidance on disposal of this book.

Primary Care Essentials
Series Editor: Georgette Eaton

The Primary Care Essentials series brings together a selection of subject-specific books which reflect the curriculum for work in primary care. These books are written specifically for the wide range of clinicians and associated professionals involved in the primary care setting and offer accessible, visual and evidence-based guidance on specific topics you may come across as part of your role.

Bringing together a multi-professional team of authors, these quick-reference resources are specifically written to support non-specialists and are ideal for double checking your knowledge whenever you need to. Whether you are a nurse, physician associate, midwife, paramedic, physiotherapist, pharmacist, or social prescriber, it provides all the essential information you need in one place, so you can feel more confident navigating your way around the breath and complexities of the primary care role.

Other titles which might be of interest:

Sexual Health
By Alyesha Proctor and Hettie Lean

Dermatology
By Sixty8 Medical

Primary Care for Paramedics
Edited by Georgette Eaton, Alyesha Proctor and Joseph St Leger-Francis

All available from Class Professional Publishing
Web: www.classprofessional.co.uk

Contents

About the Authors	vii
Acknowledgements	ix
Introduction	xi

Chapter 1: Social Prescribing, the UK Healthcare System and Primary Care — 1
- Introduction — 1
- Healthcare Challenges — 2
- Historical Context — 7
- Primary Care Context — 7
- UK Policy Influences — 9

Chapter 2: The Social Prescribing Link Worker Service — 11
- Introduction — 11
- How Social Prescribing Link Workers Work — 12
- A Week in the Life of a Social Prescribing Link Worker — 14
- The Role of the Voluntary, Community and Social Enterprise Sector — 21
- Benefits and Challenges in Social Prescribing — 22
- Social Prescribing as a Complex Intervention — 23

Chapter 3: The Social Prescribing Link Worker Workforce — 25
- Workforce Composition — 25
- Benchmark Tools and Professional Standards — 29
- Recruitment and Retention — 33

Chapter 4: Case Studies from Practice — 35
- Central Liverpool Primary Care Network (PCN) — 35
- North East London Health & Care Partnership — 37
- Health and Social Care Alliance Scotland (ALLIANCE) — 38

Conclusion and Reflections — 41

Bibliography — 43

Index — 53

About the Authors

■ National Association of Link Workers

The National Association of Link Workers (NALW) is an award winning self-governing professional and representative body, representing the pinnacle of excellence for Social Prescribing Link Workers (SPLWs). Operating independently, our membership reflects the dedication of SPLWs in providing high-quality services to patients and communities.

As the bedrock of the profession, whilst not a regulator, we spearhead standards, and advocate for the pivotal role of SPLWs in healthcare. Serving as the guiding force for SPLWs, we are also a crucial link for other professional occupational groups.

Our commitment is unwavering in ensuring safety and promoting evidence-based practices within the field. Through providing invaluable insights and intelligence, we advocate for improvements in both policy and practice related to social prescribing. The NALW serves as a unifying and professional identity for SPLWs.

■ Christiana Melam MBE

Christiana Melam is an award winning trailblazer and visionary leader in social prescribing. As the Founder and Chief Executive Officer of the National Association of Link Workers (NALW), she stands at the forefront of championing Social Prescribing Link Workers.

Christiana is the creative force behind the Annual Social Prescribing Link Worker Day, Awards, and Conference, a platform that celebrates the outstanding contributions of link workers. Her influence extends internationally, making her a revered figure in social prescribing globally.

A distinguished CEO and influencer, Christiana has earned accolades. She has also been recognised in the *Health Service Journal*'s '50 Most Influential Black, Asian, and Minority Ethnic People in Health' list for three consecutive years (2021, 2022, 2023), as well as *The Telegraph*'s prestigious

About the Authors

'100 Female Entrepreneurs to Watch List'. Acknowledged by the Mayor of London as one of the women shaping the city, she was awarded an MBE in the King's New Year's Honours List 2024 for services to social prescribing. Christiana is a sought-after keynote speaker, inspirational figure, and subject matter expert in social prescribing. With over 100 speaking engagements and numerous articles to her credit, she has become a respected voice in the field, in recognition of her outstanding contributions and subject matter expertise.

Beyond her impactful leadership, Christiana holds a Master's degree in Public Health and Health Promotion from London South Bank University, an academic, pursuing a PhD in Social Prescribing at Birmingham City University, she also teaches health and care, therapy and public health professions. Her research interests span the Social Prescribing Link Worker model, Health Inequalities, Primary and Community Health, Implementation Science, and Critical Realism. Her journey is a testament to leadership, expertise, and a profound commitment to improving healthcare systems, social prescribing and fostering community well-being.

Acknowledgements

We extend our sincere gratitude to all those whose contributions and support have played an instrumental role in the publication of this book.

Firstly, our appreciation goes to Christiana Melam MBE, Chief Executive Officer of the National Association of Link Workers who agreed to write this book on behalf of the Association.

Appreciation is extended to the Royal College of General Practitioners (RCGP) for their influential 2018 manifesto, which called for a social prescriber in every practice. This visionary stance has significantly contributed to the evolution of social prescribing.

Special thanks to the Social Prescribing Link Workers, whose dedication and tireless efforts in the field have served as the inspiration for this work. Your firsthand experiences and perspectives have added depth and authenticity to the narrative.

We would also like to express our gratitude to the organisations and individual Social Prescribing Link Workers who generously shared their case studies and practical insights (Marie Adams, Graeme Hill, Central Liverpool Primary Care Network, Health and Social Care Alliance Scotland, North East London Health & Care Partnership). Your willingness to contribute has significantly enhanced the relevance and applicability of the content.

Our heartfelt thanks to the reviewers and experts who provided valuable feedback and guidance during the development of this book. Your feedback has been helpful.

Our gratitude also goes to the broader community of healthcare professionals, policymakers, educators, researchers, people and communities who play essential roles in shaping the landscape of social prescribing. Your collective efforts are crucial in fostering positive change.

Thank you for being an essential part of this collaborative effort to shed light on the Social Prescribing Link Worker model and its impact on healthcare.

Acknowledgements

We would like to thank our readers for engaging with this book. We hope that the insights shared within these pages contribute to a deeper understanding of the Social Prescribing Link Worker model and its role in transforming healthcare.

The National Association of Link Workers

January 2024

Introduction

Social prescribing, a dynamic and evolving field within healthcare, presents itself in various models and settings. Amidst this diversity, the Social Prescribing Link Worker (SPLW) model, particularly entrenched in general practice in the UK, is the dominant model and the focus of this book. As a profession that is yet to be regulated, link workers navigate through diverse interpretations and perspectives, contributing to the confusion they face in establishing a professional identity.

This book, authored by the National Association of Link Workers, aims to provide a much-needed voice to link workers and offer insights and perspectives on social prescribing. By doing so, it illuminates the model, challenges conventional thinking, and proposes solution-focused approaches to achieving healthcare goals. Bridging policy, practice, and research, this book sets out to create a cohesive narrative for the evolving landscape of social prescribing.

■ Who Will Find This Book Insightful?

Of course, this book is about social prescribing and SPLWs, and will undoubtedly benefit those who work in these posts or aspire to. More broadly, however, this book will be useful to employers, workforce planners, educational institutions, researchers, healthcare professionals, as well as individuals interested in the Social Prescribing Link Worker model who will discover valuable insights within these pages.

■ Focus of the Book

This book is dedicated to exploring the link worker model of social prescribing, highlighting their role as a frontline non-medical healthcare worker who form an integral part of multidisciplinary teams. SPLWs are also known as Community Link Workers, Community Links Practitioners or Social Prescribers in some areas. SPLWs play a pivotal role in healthcare, and this book discusses the

Introduction

factors contributing to their success and how they help revolutionise healthcare delivery. It is written from a practice perspective.

■ Significance of the Social Prescribing Link Worker Model

Social prescribing, gaining traction among healthcare policymakers, seeks to improve health outcomes and address systemic challenges. The SPLW model challenges power dynamics within the biomedical model, representing a cultural shift in healthcare delivery that applies human rights to health.

■ Limitations and Scope

While this book provides an overview of the SPLW model, it is essential to note its limitations. Primarily focusing on social prescribing in the UK, particularly within primary healthcare, it offers a broad perspective rather than an in-depth exploration of specific local applications or exploration of various models of social prescribing. Nevertheless, local case studies in Chapter 4 enrich the understanding of the link worker model of social prescribing.

■ Collective Stance and Purpose

Recognising that social prescribing is a topic with diverse ownership interests, this book takes the bottom-up collective stance characterised in the work undertaken by the National Association of Link Workers. It is not designed to serve individual agendas but rather to empower and give voice to those trailblazing social prescribing that often feels unheard. As the first of its kind, this book serves as a starting point, offering insights and perspectives that contribute to the ongoing discourse surrounding social prescribing.

■ Book Structure

The book unfolds in four chapters, each with a distinct focus:

Chapter 1: Social Prescribing, the UK Healthcare System and Primary Care: Provides context on challenges addressed by social prescribing and explores policy drivers.

Chapter 2: The Social Prescribing Link Worker Service: Offers an overview of a SPLW service, emphasising practical aspects, operational methods, benefits, and implementation challenges.

Chapter 3: The Social Prescribing Link Worker Workforce: Focuses on the workforce, providing insights into the composition of SPLWs, benchmark tools and considerations related to recruitment and retention.

Chapter 4: Case Studies from Practice: Concludes with case studies from practice, showcasing various applications within and beyond primary care.

Overall, this book aims to contribute to the evolving field of social prescribing, acting as a catalyst for meaningful dialogue, understanding, and progress.
It is an invitation to explore and reflect, setting the stage for further discourse, research, and collaborative efforts in healthcare transformation for the public good.

CHAPTER 1

Social Prescribing, the UK Healthcare System and Primary Care

■ Introduction

Healthcare is changing, and we are dealing with challenges in managing physical, mental, and emotional health. The increase in chronic conditions, multimorbidity, an ageing population, health inequalities and the lingering mental health effects of the COVID-19 pandemic, combined with chronic workforce shortages, is a sufficient list to bring any healthcare system to a halt.

This chapter discusses several challenges within healthcare delivery that social prescribing can contribute to solving; whilst social prescribing is not the exclusive solution, nor can it independently address these challenges, it can contribute. The chapter illustrates why maintaining the current status quo is unsustainable and does not adequately meet patients' needs. It then delves into social prescribing in relation to primary care, offering background and context on why the primary care model is predominant in social prescribing and arguably the focus of the UK policy commitment in terms of social prescribing.

Social prescribing, as defined by the World Health Organization is 'a more holistic approach to healthcare, which promotes community-based integrated care and helps to demedicalise health service provision'. In the most common model, primary healthcare providers refer patients to specialised 'link workers' who collaborate with patients to identify social needs, co-design personalised plans and employ behaviour change techniques (WHO, 2022). Mercer et al. (2019) emphasises that social prescribing enhances primary care's capacity to address psychosocial and social determinants of health, while Husk et al. (2020) highlight that it systematically connects patients with non-medical community support, potentially making primary care more effective and efficient. A realist review proposed that link workers represented a vehicle for accruing social capital, which gives patients the confidence, motivation, connections, knowledge and skills to manage their own well-being

(Tierney et al., 2020). In its written submission to the Scottish Parliament Alternative pathways to primary care inquiry, NALW described social prescribing as 'non-medical treatment for non-medical determinants of health, these non-medical determinants of health include social, economic and environmental factors. By looking at these wider determinants, social prescribing is characterised by a holistic, "whole person" approach to health and wellbeing' (Scottish Parliament, 2022).

■ Healthcare Challenges

The Health Foundation's Health in 2040 report (Watt et al., 2023) predicts that a staggering 9.1 million individuals in the UK will grapple with significant illnesses by 2040, meaning 2.5 million more lives stand at a crossroads compared to 2019. At the epicentre of this health storm lies a surge of conditions – anxiety, depression, chronic pain and diabetes – casting shadows over our communities. Amid these challenges, the report highlights general practice and community-based services as the stronghold against this impending wave, with a strategy that pivots towards prevention and early intervention.

The Rise of Chronic Conditions

The healthcare challenges at the forefront of medical attention are not the same as those viewed to be most important centuries ago, or even just a few decades ago.

Multimorbidity is a term used to describe when someone has two or more long-term health conditions at the same time. The increasing prevalence of multimorbidity, a consequence of ageing populations and rising long-term conditions, poses a global public health challenge, leading to poorer outcomes, heightened utilisation of health and social care services, and escalating costs, revealing a growing awareness of the inadequacies in current healthcare service designs (Johnston et al., 2019). Furthermore, relative deprivation is another leading determinant of multimorbidity: those with the lowest wealth have a 47% higher chance of multimorbidity and a 90% higher chance of having multimorbidity with ten or more functional limitations, compared with the most affluent (Johnson et al., 2019).

This evolving category of health ailments directly correlates to the rising average lifespan (Gilbert-Johns et al., 2022); as more individuals find themselves living to older ages, new age-related diseases and conditions are developing, with one of the most common being chronic conditions. Furthermore, since the population as a whole is living longer, those with chronic conditions spend more years of their life suffering the symptoms of these conditions, requiring long-term healthcare services in order to live a life of higher quality.

Additional chronic conditions such as diabetes (NHS, 2018) and mental illness (NHS, 2017) are not related to ageing, yet their incidence in society is also rising. This evidence shows that multiple factors, beyond a rising average age, contribute to the increase in chronic conditions threatening peoples' health.

A mixed methods realist evaluation proposes that social prescribing has the potential to transform individual-level type 2 diabetes prevention by moving away from standardised, targeted and short-term strategies towards more personalised, inclusive and long-term approaches, with primary care-based social prescribing considered the most beneficial way of delivering holistic, accessible, sustained, and integrated services through collaborative efforts among practitioners, providers, and commissioners (Calderón-Larrañaga et al., 2023).

Mental Health Issues

Mental ill health is one of the most prevalent forms of illness in the UK, the economic and social cost of mental health problems in 2019/2020 is over £119 billion in England and is set to increase (Centre for Mental Health, 2021). An estimated 8.32 million identified patients received an antidepressant drug item in 2021/22 in England, which was a 5.72% increase from 2020/21 and a sixth consecutive year increase (NHSBSA, 2022).

Poor mental health often sprouts from social determinants of health and responds well to non-medical interventions. However, a complex challenge emerges when those with poor mental health and mental illness are coalesced into a single waiting list. This unintentional confluence inadvertently precipitates a decline in individuals' well-being as they await appropriate care. Addressing this issue becomes imperative to provide timely and effective care (Punton et al., 2022). Promoting a nuanced understanding of this differentiation can ensure individuals receive precisely tailored treatment that aligns with their unique circumstances. This approach effectively curtails the pervasive tendency to over-medicalise life-oriented issues and free up resources to treat severe depression and mental disorders (Doblytė, 2020). Doing so will help pave the way for a more responsive, effective, and compassionate approach to mental well-being.

With green social prescribing, there is a focused interest on the mood and health-boosting benefits offered to patients through time spent together in nature to improve mental health (Fixsen and Barrett, 2022). In England, £4 million was invested in test and learn green social prescribing projects aimed at preventing and tackling mental ill health (NHS England, 2023). There is support for the need and benefit of social prescribing to improve mental health well-being and reduce the burden of mental illness (Hassan et al., 2020).

'When it comes to mental health, there needs to be a shift from responding to mental health crises to preventing people from getting into crisis' (Christiana Melam MBE, CEO, National Association of Link Workers).

The Detriments of Loneliness

The World Health Organization (WHO, 2023) declared loneliness to be a pressing global health threat. According to the WHO, loneliness can be as dangerous for mental and physical health as smoking 15 cigarettes a day. Many underestimate how much loneliness can affect both an individual's mental and physical health. However, research into the effects of loneliness has shown that it not only increases the risk of mental health concerns such as anxiety and depression, but also the risk of physical conditions including heart disease, high blood pressure, obesity, weakened immune system, cognitive decline and even death (Cacioppo, 2014; Leigh-Hunt et al., 2017).

While these health conditions can increase a patient's need for medical attention, causing lonely people to seek primary care more frequently, these visits may not all be due to declining health. In fact, in some cases, those who are lonely visit their primary care physician in order to receive much-needed social interactions (Cruwys et al., 2018). Unfortunately, this then continues to burden the already overworked and overbooked system.

Loneliness is only becoming more prevalent, with the COVID-19 pandemic resulting in a rise of loneliness. The Office for National Statistics (2021) reported that 7.2% of the adult population feels lonely 'often' or 'always'. To combat these rising cases of loneliness, the Royal College of Psychiatrists (2021) published a report emphasising the ability of social prescribing to support mental health services, citing individuals who saw improvements in their mental well-being due to social prescribing services. Furthermore, loneliness and isolation seem to be relevant factors for suicidal ideations (McClelland et al., 2020). By improving connectedness and empowerment in patients (Galway et al., 2019), social prescribing can help reduce the risk factors for suicide.

The COVID-19 pandemic also highlighted how important being outside and in nature is for someone's mental and physical health, which is what has spurred an interest in green social prescribing. With this subset of social prescribing, there is an emphasis on linking patients to nature-based activities and interventions, with examples that include walking in nature and community gardening (NHS England, 2022).

A mixed methods evaluation of a national social prescribing programme identified social prescribing as an intervention that can be used to address loneliness; having skilled link workers who could take a service-user-led approach and having accessible activities available to signpost people to is a key to success (Foster et al., 2021).

Health Inequalities

The definition of health inequalities varies in the literature but collectively relates to systematic differences in health outcomes that are deemed avoidable, unfair and unjust, and result from an intricate interplay of socio-economic,

CHAPTER 1 • Social Prescribing, the UK Healthcare System and Primary Care

environmental and individual factors (McCartney et al., 2019). They emphasise that these differences are not random but systematic, indicating underlying causal forces. Furthermore, health inequalities are specified as being observed between different social groups. This implies that they are a population or group phenomenon rather than an individual one. The differences can manifest between categorical social groups (e.g., ethnicity, sex, nationality) or as a gradient across ranked social groups (e.g., social class, educational attainment, income bracket, area deprivation). The fundamental causes of health inequalities are unequal income, power and wealth distribution. This can lead to poverty and marginalisation of individuals and groups, influencing the distribution of wider environmental influences on health, resulting in inequalities in health outcomes (Public Health Scotland, 2021). The Fair Society, Healthy Lives (The Marmot Review) report brought great attention to the relationship between social inequalities and health inequalities and has been crucial in leading the health sector to think differently and arguably underpins the social prescribing movement (Marmot et al., 2010, Polley et al., 2020).

Health inequalities are complex and require a combination of interventions to address them. Policies targeting the reduction of income inequality, enhancement of education and improvement of employment opportunities can positively influence health outcomes (Marmot, 2010; NHS England, 2021). Collaborative community health programmes involving healthcare providers, local authorities, and community organisations have a role to play. Public health campaigns promoting healthy behaviours and addressing risk factors, such as smoking cessation, physical activity, and healthy eating, contribute to reducing health inequalities (Bickerdike et al., 2017; Featherstone et al., 2022).

The debate around health inequality largely centres around at which level and where responsibility lies and the balance between individual responsibility for health and the impact of structural factors. While some advocate for personal agency in health decisions, others emphasise the role of broader societal determinants (Marmot, 2005; Bickerdike et al., 2017). Furthermore, around the choice between universal and targeted interventions. Universal approaches aim to enhance overall societal conditions, while targeted interventions focus on specific groups at higher risk (Moffatt et al., 2017; Payne et al., 2020).

Some models of social prescribing could contribute to reduce the burden on primary care, tackle health inequalities and encourage people to make greater use of non-clinical forms of support (Bertotti et al., 2018). Social prescribing can help highlight social determinants of health affecting people's health and contributing to ongoing health concerns, as highlighted in a case study regarding a patient with respiratory health concerns living in a flat covered in mould (NALW, 2021c). When combining health inequalities with other less avoidable health concerns, such as an ageing population and comorbid health conditions, the healthcare system can take a significant hit. For instance, high-intensity use of the emergency department is estimated to cost the NHS £2.5 billion each year (British Red Cross, 2021). Furthermore, health inequalities significantly contribute to greater emergency department usage, and many visits can be avoided or better supported through social prescribing according to the British Red Cross report.

Addressing health inequality seems to be a multifaceted challenge that necessitates interventions at various levels and in combination. To enhance effectiveness, it is crucial to provide clarity and context regarding the specific focus of health inequalities targeted by each intervention, thereby bridging gaps in understanding what works for whom rather than relying on broad generalisations.

Workforce Challenges in General Practice

Over the past decade, the demand for General Practitioners (GPs) in the UK has significantly increased, posing a considerable challenge to the healthcare system. As a result, the British Medical Association (BMA) has been monitoring the workforce challenges encountered by GPs across the UK.

Wales: According to BMA (BMA 2023a) data covering the period from 2013 to 2022, the number of patients registered at GP practices in Wales witnessed a 2.9% increase, totalling 93,317. During the same period, the number of practices decreased from 470 to 386 (an 18% reduction). The equivalent number of full-time GPs decreased by 456 (21.7%) from 1,901 to 1,445. Notably, there was a rise in the average practice list size from 6,780 to 8,378 patients (23.5%), and the number of patients looked after per Full-Time Equivalent (FTE) GP increased from 1,675 to 2,210, reflecting a 32% rise. Over 80% of GPs surveyed by the BMA Cymru Wales expressed concerns about their ability to deliver quality and safe care due to overwhelming workloads, a diminishing workforce, and escalating service demands (BMA 2023b).

Scotland: Scotland is grappling with an insufficient number of GPs, with 245,193 more patients registered with GP practices in 2022 compared to 2012. Practices are compelled to cease accepting new patients, and an increasing number are closing patient lists due to insufficient resources to meet demand (BMA 2023c).

England: In England, the BMA reports that the average number of patients each GP is responsible for has surged by nearly 17% since 2015, reaching 2,260. Meanwhile the ratio of fully qualified GPs per 1,000 patients has decreased from 0.52 in 2015 to 0.44 (BMA 2023d).

Northern Ireland: General practice in Northern Ireland is in crisis, with over 17 practices surrendering their contracts since January 2023; those that remain are stretched, and GP training is undersubscribed, resulting in fewer GPs for the future.

Patients directly experience the repercussions of diminishing doctor numbers, facing longer waiting times and limited consultation durations.

CHAPTER 1 · Social Prescribing, the UK Healthcare System and Primary Care

■ Historical Context

While the idea of social prescribing is becoming more popular and discussed more frequently, especially regarding the many benefits it can provide, it is by no means a new idea.

The origins of social prescribing can be traced back to the Peckham Experiment, an investigation into the nature of health that ran from 1926 to 1950 (The Pioneer Health Foundation, 2022). The investigation took place at the Pioneer Health Centre, a location that allowed doctors to observe how families interacted in a social setting. The primary takeaway from this experiment, and the origin of social prescribing, is that the environment played a crucial role in promoting health, showing that overall health is defined as more than just the absence of disease. While this is well-known now, its discovery was ground-breaking at the time.

Over the course of the experiment, the doctors found that when people are given information about themselves and their families, they will do what they can to make the best decision for themselves and their loved ones. The doctors also found that their patients thrived when allowed to make choices about their activities and, in most cases, chose the activities that would aid their development. Regarding the community aspect, the investigation found that providing resources to a community enabled the patients to be more active in their community and work harder to better it. Unfortunately, the Second World War affected the Pioneer Health Centre resulting in it eventually closing in 1950.

Many schemes started again in the 1990s, and the Bromley by Bow Centre was established in 1984. Despite decades of use, for most of this time social prescribing was only practised in pockets, remaining primarily unnoticed by health commissioners.

■ Primary Care Context

The concept of primary healthcare (PHC) evolved during the 1970s, with The Alma-Ata Declaration of 1978 recognising primary healthcare as the key to the attainment of the goal of Health for All. Primary healthcare has been defined by the declaration at the International Conference on Primary Health Care, 1978, as:

> *Essential healthcare made accessible to individuals and families in the community, by means acceptable to them, through their full participation and at a cost that the community and the country can afford. It forms an integrated part of the country's healthcare system, of which it is the nucleus, and of the overall social and economic development of the country. Primary care is the first point of contact for healthcare for most people.*

WHO's Vision for 21st Century Primary Care

In 2018, the WHO released 'A vision for primary health care in the 21st century', outlining their current interpretation of PHC along with ways to maximise and support it. According to this most-recent document, the WHO views PHC as a whole-of-society approach aiming to equitably maximise the level and distribution of health and well-being. This definition strongly emphasises equal healthcare for all, regardless of their demographic, geographical location, financial standing, or medical condition. Furthermore, the WHO explains that maximising healthcare occurs by focusing on the preferences and needs of the individual and community as early as possible in the healthcare continuum through disease prevention and health promotion.

The three primary components of PHC that the WHO emphasises are listed in **Figure 1.1.**

The three primary components of PHC:

1. Meeting health needs through comprehensive care. This includes promotive, preventive, protective, curative, palliative and rehabilitative care.
2. Addressing broader determinants of health (economic, social, environmental, behavioural and individual characteristics).
3. Empowering communities, families and individuals to optimise their health.

The WHO vision places the central focus of healthcare improvement on individuals and communities, further showcasing the world's renewed commitment to social justice by concentrating efforts on addressing the needs of disadvantaged people. The result of this is better and more equitable healthcare for all.

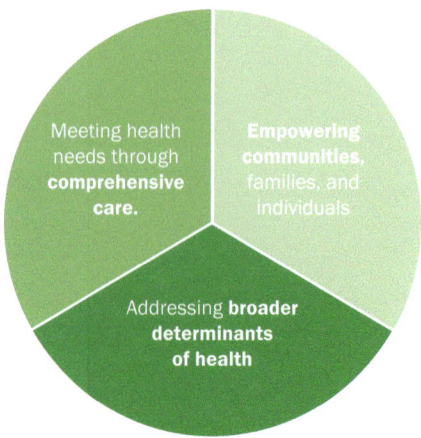

Figure 1.1 Three primary components of PHC.

Social prescribing offers a path to realising the WHO's primary healthcare vision by integrating community-based care and demedicalising complex needs (WHO, 2022), empowering individuals to address social needs, and enhancing primary care capacity to tackle psychosocial and social determinants of health which can help reduce healthcare pressures (Mercer et al., 2019; Husk et al., 2020; Tierney et al., 2020).

The Biopsychosocial Model

The model of care that encompasses three critical components of well-being, biological, psychological, and social, is the biopsychosocial (BPS) model (Engel, 1977). The very core of this model emphasises how these three factors connect.

These factors can include beliefs, trauma, coping skills and relationships, all of which are not considered when treating with the former biomedical model. Social prescribing serves to look at social and economic factors affecting mental and physical health, which allows for patients to be treated with the biopsychosocial model, a whole person approach that considers all factors affecting health and well-being. Primary care is embedded within a community. Some underserved and deprived areas traditionally lack community provisions that can improve their well-being; social prescribing can help highlight structural inequalities and community development requirements based on the unmet needs of patients.

Continuity of care is a core principle of primary care related to improved patient outcomes and reduced healthcare costs; however, patients have reported a steady decline in recent years (Tammes et al., 2021).

■ UK Policy Influences

The UK's health policies have witnessed a significant shift in the recruitment of Social Prescribing Link Workers (SPLWs) which is largely driven by healthcare challenges and patients' needs. The term 'National Health Service' (NHS) encompasses the healthcare services in the UK, with England, Scotland, Wales, and Northern Ireland individually responsible for organising and financing their respective NHS. The focus of this book is on the primary care model of social prescribing which predominantly includes a link worker, therefore this section is discussed from that perspective. SPLWs have existed in certain areas, but they gained national attention when the Royal College of General Practitioners' 2018 Manifesto advocated for every GP surgery to have access to a 'social prescriber'. This call aimed to provide support for individuals experiencing loneliness or at risk of loneliness by facilitating meaningful connections. While this was a collective stance, it is important to note that only England and Scotland's health policy directives have committed to recruitment of SPLWs as integral members of the Multidisciplinary Teams (MDT) in primary care.

Scotland and England have incorporated link workers as integral members of the Multidisciplinary Team in Primary Care, aligning with both workforce and national policy commitments. The Scottish Government introduced the Primary Care Improvement Plan (PCIP) to revamp primary care services, focusing on expanding and enhancing multidisciplinary teams to support GPs in their role as expert medical generalists, thereby enhancing patient outcomes (Scottish Government, 2023). Within the PCIP's six priority areas, the inclusion of Community Link Workers is evident, with over 300 reported to be working in primary care as of 31 March 2023. Additionally, the Scottish Government's Mental Health and Wellbeing Strategy: Delivery Plan 2023–2025 incorporates the role of link workers. In England, the NHS England Long Term Workforce plan aspires to increase the number of SPLWs to 9,000 by 2036/37 (NHS England, 2024) and they are included in several health policy national directives.

On the other hand, Wales and Northern Ireland have yet to make a nationwide commitment to the primary care workforce in terms of specific numbers of link workers. Whilst the Welsh Government's National Framework for Social Prescribing (NFfSP) is a welcome development and although the dominant model highlighted in the document is the primary care model of social prescribing, and while the document recognises that most evidence is derived from social prescribing models including a link worker or social prescribing practitioner, there is no explicit commitment to workforce numbers in the document. However, a Skills Competency Framework for social prescribing practitioners is acknowledged (Welsh Government, 2023). The SPRING Social Prescribing Project, a collaborative initiative involving Bogside & Brandywell Health Forum, the Healthy Living Centre Alliance, and Scottish Communities for Health and Wellbeing, represents a leading project for a social prescribing model incorporating a link worker role in Northern Ireland, relying on funding from The National Lottery Community Fund (SPRING, 2023). With the GP workforce challenges highlighted in the previous section with regards to Wales and Northern Ireland, it is would be interesting to investigate how social prescribing intentions are sustained without incentives or how the non link worker model is experienced in primary care.

The support within UK healthcare policy for the expansion of social prescribing with the advancement of the link worker workforce continues to grow. The unprecedented scale of investment and the rollout of link workers position the UK arguably as the global leader in social prescribing.

 For case studies from England and Scotland, refer to Chapter 4.

CHAPTER 2

The Social Prescribing Link Worker Service

■ Introduction

The Social Prescribing Link Worker (SPLW) service aims to contribute to tackling the challenges outlined in Chapter 1. This chapter provides an overview of a SPLW service regardless of the setting. It is presented from a practice standpoint, highlighting the ways link workers operate, a week in the working life, the benefits they bring and the challenges faced.

The significant advantages of social prescribing result from the role of the SPLW integrated into primary care with the support of GPs, Multidisciplinary Teams (MDTs) and multisectoral collaboration, ensuring comprehensive care and a holistic approach. Other titles, such as Community Link Worker or social prescriber, may be used interchangeably with SPLW.

SPLWs act as the bridge between the NHS and the community, functioning as integral members of the multidisciplinary team (NHS, 2022). They operate holistically and proactively, advocating for patients, service users and communities while fostering positive changes in the healthcare system at both individual and community levels. Social prescribing considers social factors influencing mental and physical health, applying the biopsychosocial model to treat patients. This comprehensive approach takes into account all factors affecting health and well-being, ensuring holistic healthcare approach.

For instance, SPLWs advocate for their patients by helping them identify holistic priorities and supporting them in accessing the most suitable services (Kiely, 2021). This empowers patients to take charge of their health and well-being, leading to better self-care and reducing the reliance on services like emergency department visits and urgent GP appointments. The concept of 'human rights in patient care', which involves applying human rights principles to patient care, including removing healthcare barriers (Cohen and Ezer, 2013), is facilitated by SPLWs.

The Social Prescribing Link Worker Model

A crucial element of a SPLW service is the involvement of Voluntary, Community, and Social Enterprise (VCSE) services. The VCSE provides the community-based support that SPLWs connect people to and will be discussed in this chapter. Whilst this chapter covers the practice elements of being a SPLW, Chapter 3 will expand on this by outlining the minimum education standards and role overview.

■ How Social Prescribing Link Workers Work

As social prescribing becomes further ingrained into healthcare and society, there is a growing need to standardise the role, scope of practice and boundaries of the SPLW, in order to increase understanding and acceptance by those they work closely with and the patients they support. With this in mind, it is beneficial to establish a model of care for the SPLW, outlining what key areas they focus on improving and the methods by which they do so.

A simplified version of how SPLWs work is as follows:

Case Finding: Those who will benefit from SPLW support are identified, or identify themselves.

Consultation: A first consultation meeting agreed upon with the person in a place that is appropriate and suitable; during the consultation, a SPLW talks about what matters to them, learns more about the upstream and downstream factors that matter the most, their values, needs, assets, obstructions and solutions they seek.

Personalised Plan: A goal-oriented and time-limited personalised support plan is **co-produced** based on what they discover together.

Solution Finding: This can take several consultations, and the needs may include four different connected issues preventing them from taking control of their health and well-being at one time. The solution can consist of multi-sectoral and multi-disciplinary team involvement and removing barriers.

Follow-up: The SPLWs review goals with the person and eventually close the casework.

Referral: There are different ways in which an SPLW receives referrals including from a GP, other healthcare professionals, self-referrals and proactive case findings.

Community Development: The model of the SPLW service recognises the role communities play in health and well-being. It acknowledges that the sustainability of behaviour change relies on whether the person feels embedded in their community and the availability of community-based support. For this reason, the role of the VCSE sector is important.

The Professional Standards Body (PRSB, 2023) Social Prescribing Information Standard in **Figure 2.1** shows the person's journey through social prescribing and the information at the different stages of their treatment and care:

CHAPTER 2 · The Social Prescribing Link Worker Service

CONTACT	CONVERSATION	INTERVENTIONS	FOLLOW-UP	OUTCOMES
Referral to link worker	**Link worker record**	**Link worker record**	**Link worker record**	**Message back to referrer and GP**

• Person demographics
• GP details
• Referral details (to/from)
• Presenting needs
• Risks & Safeguarding
 	
Plus supporting information via referral or via shared care record
• About me
• Individual requirements
• Care & support plan
• Relevant problems
• Social context
	• Meetings details
	• Care & support plan including:
	  • Needs
	  • Strengths
	  • Goals
	  • Actions and activities
	• Updates to person details
	• Meetings summary
		• Referrals
		• Signposting
		• Attendance
			• Meetings details
			• Progress notes
			• Outcome assessments
				• Consent to share
				• Summary
				• Actual Needs
				• Actions & activities
				• Assessments
				• Updated person details
				• Plan and requested actions for GP/ professionals & person

Figure 2.1 The social prescribing journey.

Source: Professional Record Standards Body: https://theprsb.org/standards/social-prescribing-standard/. Reproduced with permission.

13

The Social Prescribing Link Worker Model

■ A Week in the Life of a Social Prescribing Link Worker

Marie and Graham share what a week is like!

Marie's Story

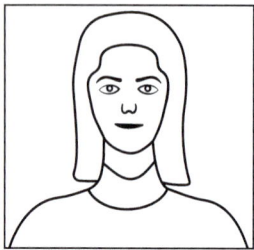

My name is Marie, I am a social prescriber based in a GP practice. I work with patients of all ages and my mentor encourages me to develop my role.

Monday

Morning tasks include:

Administrative tasks including jobs and emails sent over the weekend.

Face-to-Face (F2F) with a patient who has previously attempted suicide but was found and saved in time. We chat and explore new ways of working. The patient recently saw a GP who has prescribed medication and she is now working with a trained counsellor who is able to offer support from past trauma.

Share progress via a note to the GP describing how our intervention has had such a positive outcome; the patient is now able to leave home on her own, has returned to work on a phased return and was smiling, something she couldn't do seven months ago.

F2F patient who is coping with bereavement and grief after the loss of a relative has had an impact on his well-being. We discuss how to fill the void left from his caring responsibilities. He has made new friends and taken up a couple of hobbies. He is also letting out the neighbour's new puppy each day whilst they are at work and can spend over an hour playing in the garden together.

Lunch for 30 minutes

Afternoon tasks include:

Review emails

F2F patient who is concerned that her bipolar will be managed by Primary Care (GP) and not Community Mental Health (CMH) who have always dealt with any changes to her medication in the past. I make a note to speak with her GP and contact CMH to see what processes can be put in place to this effect.

14

Patient has cancelled so I use the time to follow up on the four patients on my clinic list.

F2F with a family completing an ADHD (Attention Deficit Hyperactivity Disorder) questionnaire to refer to CAMHS (Children and Adolescent Mental Health Service); I scan completed form and ask the GP to refer to CAMHS. I could do the referral but, in this instance, there are some specific issues that I would like the GP to be made aware of and bring to CAMHS' attention. I was able to share county CAMHS website and resources and the 'Back to Basics' programme with the family.

Tuesday

Morning tasks include:

Contact new patients. In total I have contacted twelve via text either sharing contact information from the Level 2 weight management and exercise programme, refer to Mind Decider 4 – six-week programme and/or send them a date for a face-to-face appointment.

Meeting with manager to discuss how things are going with work and personally. Last year I was quite ill from a mixture of a bad cold, tiredness and overwork. My colleagues and managers are incredibly supportive and understand that I put everything into supporting my patients, because I cannot help but be me. We also discuss the number of new referrals in the past month which was 155 (This can range from 80–180 per month).

Any leave planned is also discussed so as not to interrupt patient care.

We also cover the projects that I am involved with including developing new virtual PPG (Patient Participation Group) at my surgery, Mental Health Transformation (MDT) meetings, NALW (National Association of Link Workers) training and presentations, creating opportunities for public health Hampshire and CAMHS to review messages and publications.

Lunch: NALW member meeting to find out about new developments. I have my lunch at the same time.

Afternoon tasks include:

Catching up on internal and external emails, EMIS Tasks and allocation of new patients and teams messages and actions. There are several ways in which people communicate and I must ensure that all messages are replied to promptly; however, it is not always possible as responding to people who are caring for loved ones need a thoughtful reply. I also must consider that there is only one of me and 11,000 patients in our surgery.

F2F with a new patient who is struggling with depression. Her employer has not been very supportive and has stopped her pay. Her union have not done very much or offered any support. A nurse has referred her as she feels I will be able to listen and refer her on to more supportive organisations who will be able to help. I was able to have a conversation with Citizens Advice and arrange an appointment for her to get advice on employment law. I was able to offer support and encouragement by meeting with her and referred her to a new supportive sleep programme she was not aware of; I also allowed her to talk and vent about her situation in a safe and confidential space.

F2F appointment with a patient who I have tried to arrange several meetings with but does not attend. Unfortunately, they did not attend today either. I used this time for administration and contacted six patients that I have to follow up as well as 13 new patients.

Wednesday

Morning tasks include:

Patient cancelled so I will continue with my two follow-up patients and six new patients, triaging and arranging appointments and sharing information as needed.

I have my weekly meeting with my mentor (clinical supervisor) where we discuss any patients that I have. We also discuss any of his patients for whom he needs me to be aware of any background information. We have worked together for over two years and during that time he has allowed my role to develop and grow. He has ensured through his training that I have knowledge and am confident within my patient consultations. He has explained subjects such as pain management and how medication works, along with how certain departments work such as mental health services, diagnose and discharge and the role of primary care. I now see a wide variety of children and families where CAMHS are unlikely to engage and offer alternative contacts. His support and championing of me has ensured my role is embedded within the surgery.

Home visit – the patients are housebound and elderly. I have a carer's pack that I share which includes all the information needed to support people's independence at home. Although they are reluctant, I am able to encourage the patients to have a Social Services home assessment. I encourage them to find out about free resources and if they still are not interested, they can decide not to move forwards at any time. Support is usually needed with personal care and help with meals, so care can often be planned around one visit; it doesn't have to be seven days a week if family and friends are able to help with meals and a wash. Family members do not usually want to be involved with personal care but there are other ways to help. There are many other things that support is needed for such as shopping and just visiting for a coffee.

Health Inequalities meeting – this is a bi-monthly meeting for an hour to discuss progress of our annual project. This year the annual project relates to carers' access to surgeries and information to support them and the person they care for. We have been attending local community events that promote our role and handing out carer's packs. We have also been working with surgery staff to identify carers and new carers and posting carers packs to them.

Lunch: TARGET training event for three hours – PCN (Primary Care Network) is delivering a well-being session for the whole team, and afterwards we are going bowling.

Thursday

Morning tasks include:

Home visit – an elderly patient who struggles with her mobility and hearing. Before she became a widow her husband paid all the bills and insisted there was always money in the account. Attendance Allowance pays for a cleaner, however she does not want to release any of her savings to pay for further support. As a patient of over three years, I have previously taught her to order shopping online and she is independent, but frail. Whilst I have offered many alternatives to leave the house she is adamant that she is okay.

Follow up on six patients and emails.

Lunch: 30 minute lunch in staff room as it is important to meet surgery colleagues and meet face-to-face rather than just through screen messages.

Afternoon tasks include:

Library visit to support a lady in joining the local library. We will use a computer to sign in to her Universal Credit account as we are currently doing this once a week at the GP surgery. She became homeless this year and was sleeping outside. Several events lead up to this situation, but the key factor was that she worked in an elderly hospital ward and the number of deaths during and following COVID-19 took its toll. Unfortunately, her employer did not understand the effect it had on her. I have been working for nine months with this lady who is now housed in over 55s' accommodation, is claiming Universal Credit and volunteering once a week in order to develop her confidence and conversation skills. We are working with Jobcentre Plus and the local college to develop her computer skills and next year we hope she will be skilled enough to apply for a local job as there are currently a few gaps. The employment agency is pleased she is being pro-active and learning new skills and is giving her the time needed for this.

I return to the surgery and work on the four follow-up patients and outstanding 20 new patients.

Friday

Morning tasks include:

Two hours for weekly peer support and the four PCN social prescribers meet up to discuss new groups. They learn from supporting patients and each other with difficult cases. If this time wasn't built into our week, we would be isolated and working in silos as we all work in our own separate surgeries. Last week we also had our monthly social prescriber team meeting.

Presentation from a hot meal supplier in the community and taste testing. I give my over 65-year-old patients information on this supplier as a healthy choice, so they have more choices than supermarket ready meals as it has vegetables and healthy nutrients included in the dish.

Lunch: 12:30pm had lunch with SP colleagues at local coffee shop.

Afternoon tasks include:

Friday afternoons are used to catch up on administration and previously unavailable patients for that week.

Plan next week's appointments and information I may need to share including my flyer with my work email and the surgery phone number on. If I am talking to someone who may need a quicker response, I will share my work phone number to text and call them back.

General Reflections:

I am always humbled when a patient thanks me for the support I have given them or when they feedback on something I had told them, and they are now doing it.

My surgery colleagues tell me they couldn't do my job as my patients need time to work through and they haven't the patience I seem to have. I will never forget a nurse telling me: 'I know the referrals I make to you will be taken seriously and not discharged until you have done everything to help them'.

My clinical supervisor has told me many times my passion for social prescribing is infectious and full of enthusiasm. Once, whilst I was on a course one of the participants said: 'I wish I was a patient at your surgery and could see you'.

My line manager has told me she doesn't know how I do all that I do, and it is exhausting listening to what I am doing for my patients and promoting the benefits of social prescribing. She always thanks me for all the hard and positive work that I am doing.

Key Takeaways:

Until I see a patient and have a conversation, I do not know what we will be discussing or the progress they have made. I prepare information to share and takeaway, but never pre-empt the appointment.

Time goes so quickly, and this can be frustrating, but as I tell my patients it's always one step at a time. I can only work on one patient at a time.

Don't feel guilty for working late or opening the laptop at the weekend, but only do this in moderation! Social prescribers give so much to their patients, they need you to follow your own advice.

Adapt your clinic to work for you. As long as the slots have a patient's name in, I do follow up with patients and they can be followed up from one month to two years later, depending on the patient and the support they needed (as not everyone has someone to help them).

Our annual target of 250 patients set by the NHS allows us the time to spend with new patients and I allow a two-hour slot for our initial chat, writing up of notes and any actions. The follow-up slot will be up to an hour, but don't be afraid to book longer if they need it or you are supporting them to go to a group or employment agency. I have learnt that our patients need more support and if we offer it, we need to be pro-active and deliver it!

Graeme's Story

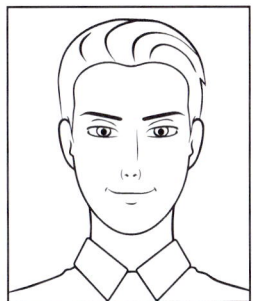

My name is Graeme, I'm a GP practice based SPLW. I work in three practices and work with people aged 18+. I have been doing my job for four years.

Monday

- Based in the GP practice for the day.
- A mixture of telephone and face to face appointments.
- Assisting with completing Universal Credit form.
- Supporting person into social settings following diagnosis of autism.
- Assisting person who has hoarding difficulties at home.
- Triage. Meet with social prescribing colleagues online to discuss and allocate referrals received from clinicians.

Tuesday

- Based in another GP practice.
- A mixture of telephone and face to face appointments.
- Attend SPLW champion peer support group. Discuss national and regional developments.
- Home visit to assist a lady to purchase a mobility scooter.
- Telephone appointment for a lady who wants more exercise activities.
- Referral to Leisure Trust who provide physical activities.
- Referral to Heywood Middleton & Rochdale Circle service specialising in reducing isolation for people 50+.

The Social Prescribing Link Worker Model

Wednesday

- Based in a third GP practice.
- Assist client with PIP (Personal Independence Payment) form completion.
- Face-to-face appointment with a lady who is a victim of domestic abuse.
- Appointment with client who is feeling very isolated and wants to explore new activities.
- Attend online training in strengths-based conversations.
- Attend MDT meeting regarding a lady who is in long term support to build independence in the community.

Thursday

- In the community. Project based work.
- Development schemes linked with GP practices that provide safe places for people to reengage back in the community.
- Bike library and allotment projects.
- Draw up funding bid to financially support projects.
- Open bank account for the community group and constitute community group.
- Submit monitoring and evaluation forms to grant providers.
- Meeting with Public Health directorate regarding promoting social prescribing in the borough.

Friday

- In the community. Project based work.
- Green Prescribing Allotment programme. Meet with and support volunteers on the programme.
- Administration. Catch up on recording appointments.
- Attend conference and present to Royal Pharmaceutical Society on case studies and role of social prescribing.
- Complete NALW Level 5 Social Prescribing question on accredited paper.

General Reflections:

A man who is involved in the green prescribing programme said that without the opportunity to engage in this he would have been just sat at home feeling depressed and not having the motivation to get out: 'I have skills. I'm very good with wood but I wasn't able to enjoy those skills. I built a raised planter for the project. This has given me a sense of purpose. I knew I was declining and really needed to do something'. This highlights the rewards of the SPLW role and the difference it makes to individuals and communities.

Key Takeaways:

Key learning is the importance of people having a sense of purpose and belonging. People lose the strength and motivation to leave their homes and be with people. Working in conjunction with clinicians in this area can turn a person's life around.

Is the SPLW Role Prescriptive?

> Not at all: It's about Patient Empowerment and Enablement

The SPLW and patient interaction is reconfigured from a traditional clinical approach and offers a more relational approach. Patients co-produce their personalised care plan, and the SPLW harnesses from the already existing knowledge people have of the issues they face taking a strengths-based approach. Demonstrative of the changing power dynamics between patients and health providers is the debated terminology related to social prescribing. The term 'prescribing', traditionally a clinical term, is used in this context where SPLWs do not prescribe but rather guide patients in identifying the most suitable solutions for addressing the health needs of specific individuals.

Marie and Graeme's descriptions of a week in the life of a SPLW demonstrates the variability and complexity of the role and the continuity of care element. With SPLWs embedded in primary care, it enables GPs to have a holistic view of what is going on for their patients and can help jointly come up with a better management plan (NALW, 2022d).

■ The Role of the Voluntary, Community and Social Enterprise Sector

The support and growth of the voluntary, community and social enterprise (VCSE) sector is vital to the success of the SPLW model. The VCSE comprises independent and self-governing organisations that provide community-based solutions and activities to better the community through promoting economic, social, cultural, or environmental objectives for health promotion and improving care outcomes (NHS Confederation, 2020). These ideals align with the social prescribing goal of increasing prevention and self-care. SPLWs can also raise awareness of the work the VCSE sector completes, which further displays to healthcare professionals the benefits of community services for patients and the many available offerings (Tierney et al., 2020).

The VCSE and small peer support groups play a crucial role in behaviour change and sustaining behaviour. Peer support groups allow people to seek guidance and support from others who have been, or are currently, in the same position as them, and they have a role in sustaining behaviour. An important measure of social prescribing success often overlooked, could be whether there is an increasing number of peer support groups available in the community. In addition, some fully funded SPLW services may have microgrants to support community initiatives and fill gaps in service provision. Social prescribing is a complex intervention, and funding has not always been made available for the entire patient journey, including SPLWs and the community development component (VCSE).

■ Benefits and Challenges in Social Prescribing

Social prescribing is at the forefront of healthcare innovation, garnering growing interest in expanding its practices in primary care and beyond due to its potential and benefits. However, challenges need to be addressed.

The benefits of social prescribing are varied and generally centre around a holistic approach to health, patient-centred care, out-of-hospital care, preventive health strategy, mental health benefits, supporting social determinants and reduced healthcare utilisation.

In their 2023 study, Pollard et al., found that social prescribing offers significant help for individuals with long-term health conditions. However, link workers experienced challenges in embedding social prescribing in an established primary care and voluntary sector landscape. The study stresses the importance of careful implementation of social prescribing within primary care to effectively support those facing disadvantages. Mercer et al., (2019) emphasise that social prescribing enhances primary care's capacity to address psychosocial and social determinants of health, while Husk et al., (2020) highlight that it systematically connects patients with non-medical community support, potentially making primary care more effective and efficient. A realist review proposed that link workers represented a vehicle for accruing social capital, which gives patients the confidence, motivation, connections, knowledge and skills to manage their own well-being (Tierney et al., 2020).

Challenges to social prescribing include a lack of rigorous evidence, standardisation challenges, potential medicalisation of social issues, equity and access concerns, and variability in outcomes. The National Association of Link Workers (NALW, 2021a) report underscores challenges encountered by Social Prescribing Link Workers. Foremost among these is a pervasive lack of understanding regarding their roles and boundaries (40%), closely followed by a dearth of adequate support (38%). The seamless integration of social prescribing into primary care is hindered by oversight of General Practitioners' roles and organisational adaptations (The King's Fund, 2022). One in three SPLWs expressing intentions to resign (NALW, 2020b) poses a potential threat to the sustainability of social prescribing.

Most recently, in 2023, Unison trade union passed a motion calling for standardisation of education and support for social prescribing (UNISON, 2023). Similarly, GPs' Local Medical Committee passed a motion calling for adequate supervision provision and resourcing for all additional roles in general practice, also known as ARRS (this includes SPLWs). Education and supervision standards will be covered in Chapter 3.

The impact of budget cuts on the VCSE sector, vital for social prescribing, is significant. Estimates of £4.3 billion from March to May 2020 led to the dissolution of many organisations (UK Research and Innovation). SPLWs report that a decline in VCSE offered services makes their role more challenging, similar to a GP running out of essential medication.

Acknowledging the complexity of social prescribing, bridging the gap between research, policy, and practice is crucial for its meaningful advancement. Still in its infancy and evolving, social prescribing requires more research. Future research would benefit from comprehensive intervention developmental processes, with reference to appropriate theory, alongside long-term follow-up outcome assessment, using treatment fidelity strategies and a focus on the principle of person-centred care (Cooper et al., 2022).

NALW's strategic priorities, periodically updated, provide valuable insights for researchers interested in this subject. Current focal points include various SPLW models, access disparities, referral pathways, integrated team working, education frameworks, caseload dynamics, supervision types, pay structures and more.

> For further information and updated priorities, visit the NALW website at: https://www.nalw.org.uk

■ Social Prescribing as a Complex Intervention

An intervention such as a SPLW's, might be considered complex because of properties of the intervention itself, such as the number of components involved, the range of behaviours targeted, expertise and skills required by those delivering and receiving the intervention; the number of groups, settings, or levels targeted; or the permitted level of flexibility of the intervention or its components (Skivington et al., 2021).

Chapter 1 laid the foundation for the premise of social prescribing. However, when it comes to collecting outcomes of social prescribing interventions, there is currently no standardised approach to measuring these outcomes, and the method by which data is collected can vary based on the reason for collecting the data, such as for formal research or as a part of routine monitoring as alluded to in the challenges section. There also needs to be more clarity between outputs and outcomes. There is room for continued outcome reporting in specific areas to address challenges in evaluating various social prescribing benefits. For example, (Polley et al., 2022) found that very few studies focused on the effect of social prescribing on wider determinants of health such as skills and education, instead focusing more on health outcomes. At the time of writing, there are also no studies that have reported results for specific determinants of health such as legal, crime, or welfare issues.

The Medical Research Council framework for developing and evaluating complex interventions guidance (Skivington et al., 2021), highlights four main phases of research: intervention development or identification, for example from policy or practice, feasibility, evaluation, and implementation.

At each phase, the guidance suggests that six core elements should be considered, (see **Figure 2.2**).

1. How does the intervention interact with its context?
2. What is the underpinning programme theory?
3. How can diverse stakeholder perspectives be included in the research?
4. What are the main uncertainties?
5. How can the intervention be refined?
6. Do the effects of the intervention justify its cost?

Figure 2.2 Complex intervention guidance.

Social prescribing has to be understood as a complex intervention impacting individuals, communities, GP and MDTs; data collection and the role of SPLW must be standardised (NALW, 2023a; NALW, 2021a), so that there is clarity, and the whole patient journey is considered in the evaluation. Suppose the published Social Prescribing Information Standard (PRSB, 2022) discussed in Chapter 3 is implemented. In that case, it will enable consistency in recording information for the whole patient journey. Further more, Evers et al's (2024) scoping review found theories were mainly used to interpret qualitative findings, with one for hypothesis testing and none for the development of the social prescribing programme. Addressing these challenges in conjunction with the workforce challenges highlighted in Chapter 3 will allow for a better understanding and implementation of the primary care SPLW model.

CHAPTER 3

The Social Prescribing Link Worker Workforce

Chapter 2 covered the Social Prescribing Link Worker (SPLW) service, including the challenges the workforce faces to reach their full potential and offer the benefits seen in the growing evidence base. This chapter will examine the SPLW workforce composition, careers, professional practice, standards, recruitment and retention.

■ Workforce Composition

As of February 2023, NHS England reported 2,577 SPLWs just within England (NHS England, 2023), with 308 reported to be working in primary care in Scotland as of 31 March 2023 (Scottish Government, 2023). In the absence of a mandatory register of SPLWs, it is impossible to accurately report the number of link workers; NALW is not a regulator and positions itself as a voluntary professional and representative body. However, as discussed in Chapter 1, there are initiatives to increase the outreach of social prescribing throughout the UK, primarily through increasing the number of link workers.

The SPLW workforce come from a range of backgrounds. The National Association of Link Workers (NALW) through a series of surveys and intelligence, gathered information regarding the SPLW workforce and their route into this role, such as:

- Most SPLWs have a background in healthcare, social care, or VCSE before becoming a link worker.
- The SPLWs who were surveyed gained their experience, skills, and knowledge from various frontline-facing jobs, including those in health and social care, charities, local councils and other public and private sectors.

- The qualifications of surveyed SPLWs varied, with some not having any degree at the time of entry into the field to those who hold up to a Master's degree.
- Personal attributes and experience were viewed as important.

The NALW's career pathway research (NHS, 2023) highlighted as follows:

Entry routes into SPLW role:

- Progression from another role
- Upskill training
- Volunteering
- Personal attributes
- Qualification in a relevant subject
- Experience
- Plus, experience relevant to the role.

Previous experience, knowledge and skills reported by respondents:

A range of learned experience, skills and knowledge gained from various frontline client-facing jobs in health and social care, charities, local councils and other public and private sectors, such as:

- Social services
- Housing, mental health and homelessness support
- Care coordinator or other PCN roles
- Nutrition, health and fitness roles
- Community development and partnerships
- Social welfare and advice work
- Domiciliary care.

Qualifications of SPLW respondents included Master's/Bachelor's Degrees, NVQs, Diplomas in:

- Education
- Social work
- Lifestyle
- Community development
- Coaching
- Counselling
- Management
- Health and social care
- Public health.

Roles people reported moving on to:

- Progression with the SP team to senior, lead SPLW
- Managerial role within the service or another service
- Specialist SPLW role
- Community development

- Project management
- SPLW setting up a new service in another locality
- SPLW for another service with better pay and working conditions
- Remain as an SPLW working for same organisation
- Return to previous role
- AHP roles, or assistant AHP roles
- Entrepreneurship
- Lifestyle roles.

Portfolio Career

In recent times, the NALW has created portfolio career paths to enhance the retention of SPLW, providing an alternative to those who seek variation and trailblaze professional experience where the necessary skills can be developed to build the profession (see **Figure 3.1**). This includes:

– Educational Assessor
– Professional or Educational Supervisor
– Peer Researcher

While the diverse backgrounds and different qualifications of SPLWs entering this new unregulated profession is a strength as it allows equal opportunity, it also shows a need for standardised, flexible entry routes, codes of practice, and education standards that unite all SPLWs, regardless of their pathway into the field, to make the profession sustainable and reduce risks as they are frontline healthcare workers managing caseloads. The varied backgrounds and qualifications of SPLWs in this emerging, unregulated field offer both strengths and challenges. While they provide equal opportunity, there's a pressing need for standardised entry routes, codes of practice, and education standards to ensure professional cohesion and sustainability. This is crucial given their frontline role in healthcare, where they manage caseloads and face inherent risks. There is no denying that growing the SPLW workforce is beneficial for patients, communities, and healthcare; but it also raises the risk of letting new and existing link

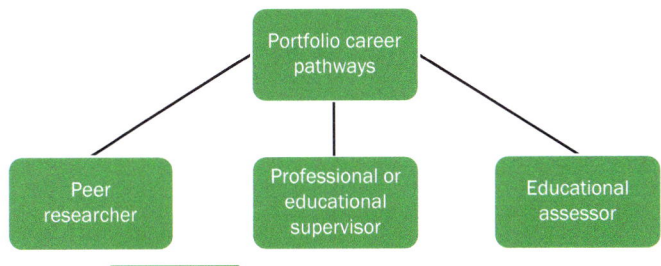

Figure 3.1 Career paths for SPLWs.

workers being inadequately deployed, whether regarding the education they receive pertaining to the role or the support (or lack thereof) they receive within their job.

In 2021, over 70% of SPLWs who responded to the NALW's survey supported regulation of the role mainly due to the lack of adequate support, training, supervision, pay, working conditions and role variations. To ensure this workforce is appropriately prepared at all stages of their career to complete their essential functions, specific professional standards and benchmark tools must be in place to set universal expectations for the roles, abilities, and requirements of the SPLW. Furthermore, in 2023, NALW introduced accredited registration options and qualifications and in 2024 renewed calls for regulation of the role to reduce variation and ensure adequate training, supervision and support.

Establishing consistent education standards alongside adaptable pathways to demonstrate competence, such as qualifications, portfolios, and apprenticeships, is crucial. Individuals become SPLWs with varied backgrounds and goals, some specializing from the start while others transition. As a specialised field, SPLWs adhere to specific codes of practice and educational benchmarks. Thus, any entry route should align with these standards.

Competency in educational standards can be attained through evidence portfolios or formal qualifications. The importance of uniform education is underscored by the requirement to present evidence portfolios or qualifications during the application process for NALW accreditation, serving as a benchmark for educational standards.

Types of Social Prescribing Link Workers

SPLWs can work in various settings, such as:

- Primary care
- Community care
- Secondary care
- Other non-healthcare settings.

They may also focus on specific populations or unmet needs, such as:

- Adults
- Children and young people
- Mental health
- Maternal health
- Armed forces
- Carers
- Migrant groups
- Homeless health
- Dementia
- Cancer.

CHAPTER 3 • The Social Prescribing Link Worker Workforce

■ Benchmark Tools and Professional Standards

The NALW Code of Practice, Education Standards, supervision and endorsed Professional Record Standards Body Social Prescribing Information Standard (PRSB, 2022) benchmark tools support the SPLW workforce and employers to ensure patients and communities receive high-quality SPLW model services.

Codes of Practice

The Code of Practice for the SPLW sets the core standards expected of a high-quality social prescribing practice. Not only does this provide guidelines and structure for the SPLW so that they understand their role, but NALW has also reported that their members, patients and public members place greater trust in a professional whose work is underpinned by a code of practice (NALW, 2022a). As such, following the SPLW Code of Practice is crucial for increasing trust and confidence in the service. It was first published in 2019 and is in two parts: one for SPLWs and one for employers.

Code of Practice for Employers of Social Prescribing Link Workers

As an employer, the Code of Practice for Employers of Social Prescribing Link Workers sets out responsibilities for ensuring SPLWs are competent and supported enough to achieve the standards required (see **Figure 3.2**).

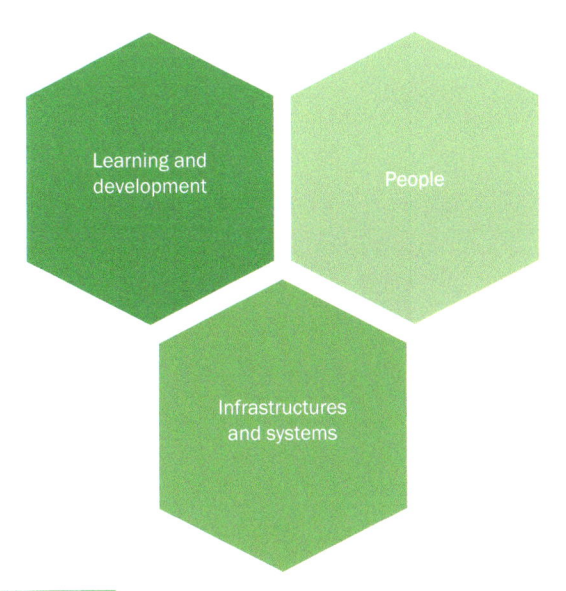

Figure 3.2 Code of practice for employers of SPLWs.

The Social Prescribing Link Worker Model

Employers are required to:
- Make sure people are suitable and are the right fit for the social prescribing model.
- Have the infrastructures and systems in place to support SPLWs to meet the Code of Practice.
- Provide learning and development opportunities to enable social prescribing workers to enhance their skills, knowledge and build resilience.

Code of Practice for Social Prescribing Link Workers

As a SPLW, the Code of Practice for Social Prescribing Link Workers sets out responsibilities for meeting the standards and ensuring professional competence (see **Figure 3.3**).

Promote the holistic well-being, rights and interests, of individuals and carers.

Build and maintain the trust and confidence of people who use services and carers.

Promote the independence of people who use services while protecting them, as far as possible, from danger and harm.

Act with integrity, uphold public trust and confidence in the SPLW profession.

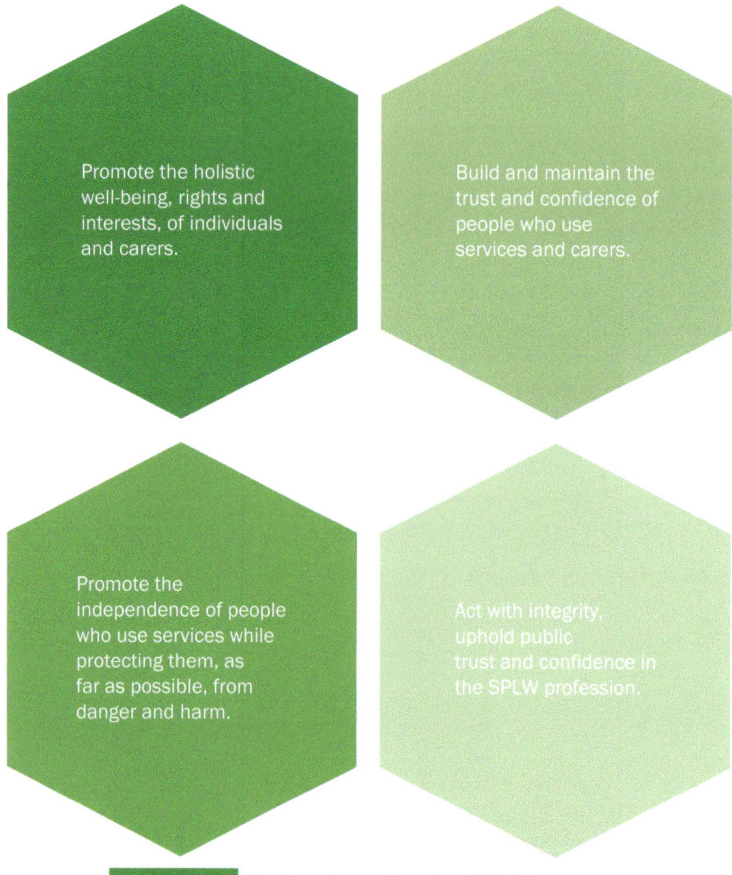

Figure 3.3 Code of practice for SPLWs.

CHAPTER 3 • The Social Prescribing Link Worker Workforce

Social prescribing link workers are required to:
- Promote the holistic well-being, rights and interests, of individuals and carers.
- Build and maintain the trust and confidence of people who use services and carers.
- Promote the independence of people who use services while protecting them, as far as possible, from danger and harm.
- Act with integrity, uphold public trust and confidence in the SPLW profession.

A detailed description of each code can be found in the Code of Practice for Employers of Social Prescribing Link Workers and Social Prescribing Link Workers as released by the NALW (NALW, 2022a). These are subject to review and updated versions can be found on the NALW's website.

Education Standards

The NALW Education Standards for Social Prescribing Link Workers (NALW, 2022b) identifies the minimum level of knowledge and skills expected of link workers to practice confidently and independently. The Education Standards are based upon the Code of Practice for link workers, and as such, they can aid professional practice and support any national statutory and/or local guidance.

The Education Standards consist of five sections, as laid out by the NALW. See **Figure 3.4**.

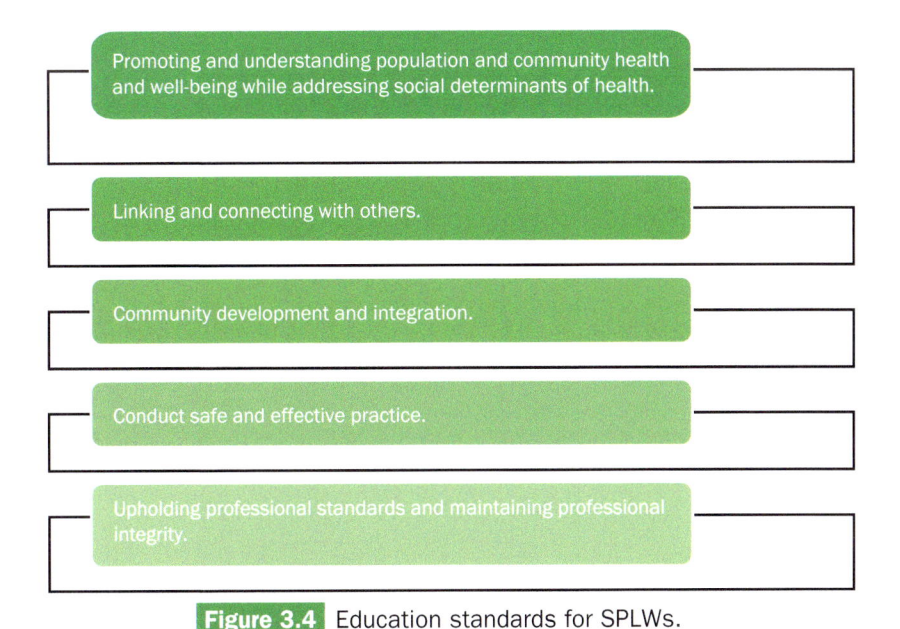

- Promoting and understanding population and community health and well-being while addressing social determinants of health.
- Linking and connecting with others.
- Community development and integration.
- Conduct safe and effective practice.
- Upholding professional standards and maintaining professional integrity.

Figure 3.4 Education standards for SPLWs.

For a deeper exploration of the Education Standards, the learning outcomes for each section can be found in Education Standards for Social Prescribing Link Workers (NALW, 2022b) and online.

Supervision

Supervision is a formal activity crucial for helping SPLWs to develop and feel supported as they complete their role designations. Furthermore, there are different types of supervision, and each offers benefits in addressing the challenges that keep the benefits of social prescribing from being realised. For example, one type of supervision may ensure that the link worker feels adequately integrated into the team, while another type holds the SPLW's professional development to the highest standard. The goal of supervision is to help the link worker overcome any difficulties they are facing and develop and reflect on their practice, which is why regular supervision is crucial for SPLW success. Additionally, supervision must be readily accessible and flexible to the needs of the individual, and the complexity of their role. Supervision is not just the responsibility of one and is not completed in just one format.

> The NALW, on behalf of NHS England, collaborated to develop short films, which further detail different methods of supervision for those interested in exploring the different types of supervision, and what they entail, in more depth (NALW, 2022g).

Types of Supervision

Workplace Supervision

(a) Line management supervision: As standard as per employer's guidelines.

(b) Clinical supervision: Supervision to support complexity, ensuring practising within the scope of practice, patient safety, guidelines and pathway. This type of supervision is carried out by an appropriate clinician and is usually determined by the service type and their regulatory requirements. For example, if you are a GP practice or hospital SPLW, you may or may not require this type of supervision.

Professional Supervision

Supervision to support development, competence and reflection is carried out by someone who understands the job of SPLWs, ethics and education standards (ideally a competent SPLW or a competent educator). Benchmarks tools such as education standards or code of practice can be used as support tools and to identify developmental needs.

Format

Supervisions may be carried out on an individual basis or as a group.

Frequency and Records

Supervision is a formal activity and should be readily available; there should be a supervision record with a monthly minimum frequency.

> NALW's supervisor training standards provide guidance on supervision and minimum training requirements and is available online (NALW, 2023b).

Social Prescribing Information Standard

The Professional Record Standards Body (PRSB, 2022) published the Social Prescribing Information Standard to enable the sharing and recording of information for the whole patient journey, from initial referral, throughout the period of social prescribing and the reply to the referrer and GP at its conclusion.

According to PRSB, the standard supports the recording and sharing of information including:

- The information required to support the conversations between the link worker and the person.
- Information to support people, to show their healthcare is joined-up and avoid repetition of their story.
- Information that can be shared with the person themselves, their family or carer.
- Summary information back to the referrer and GP for the person's overall record.
- Information for secondary uses, such as understanding the scale and effectiveness of social prescribing services, planning and population health.

> This also links to **Figure 2.1** on p. 13 which shows the person's journey through social prescribing and this standard applies in practice.

■ Recruitment and Retention

The NALW published a study on the knowledge, skills, experiences and support needs of link workers (NALW, 2019a). Within this study, the NALW conducted a survey on link workers which revealed areas where SPLWs require extra support, such as training, peer networking, and clinical supervision while working with a variety of service users who have a range of conditions or complex issues. Additional surveys completed by the NALW (2019a) highlighted a need by link workers for reflective practice and independent peer supervision. Rhodes' (2021) study supported the assertion that working as a SPLW is a complex and demanding role and subsequently needs adequate training and support.

Acknowledging the areas where SPLWs feel they need more support to properly complete their job roles is crucial for retaining current workers. In fact, one of the most common complaints among SPLWs is a lack of support even as they struggle to complete their work, which can leave many considering a different profession. A 2020 survey conducted by the NALW revealed that 29% of SPLWs are considering resigning within a year because of a lack of clinical supervision and/or support. These results are not surprising when the survey also revealed that 61% of the participants had no clinical supervision, and 11% had no supervision at all (NALW, 2020b). A scoping review identified priority areas of focus for practitioners and researchers, to include explorations of staff training and supervision (Sandhu et al., 2022).

Employers need to understand the role they are recruiting into, the outcomes they seek, and what is required to deliver those outcomes. The code of practice for employers is a guide for employers in conjunction with the education standards. Moore et al., 2023 suggest that future research should track the development of social prescribing and assess how the national push towards homogeneity, professionalisation and uniform protocols aligns with service users' needs. To maintain a competent and robust SPLW workforce, it is crucial to provide them with the required support, education, and development. Therefore, the delivery of the desired social prescribing benefits relies on who you are able to recruit and retain. Patient accounts consistently suggest that the link worker is key to the success of the pathway; however, they must be recruited, trained and supported with a clear understanding of the demands of this complex role (Frostick and Bertotti, 2021).

The role of SPLWs is multifaceted, encompassing clinical support, public health and psychological well-being depending on the model. Reflecting the diversity and complexity of their responsibilities, appropriate salary levels necessitate a comprehensive job evaluation. Employers are also encouraged to conduct a local job evaluation of the role to determine the appropriate pay, as pay issues are a common reason for resignation or moving to another organisation offering better pay according to NALW's insights.

Disparities in salaries exist, with some SPLWs reporting low salaries and limited progression opportunities. This is despite NHS England's guidance indicating that SPLWs may earn 'around £27,000 per annum', equivalent to a band 5 NHS worker (Moore et al., 2023). Another study reported a broader salary range of £16,000–£32,000 (Wallace et al., 2021). This variability is compounded by different models and levels of social prescribing.

Additionally, exploring the impact on recruitment, job retention and job satisfaction for SPLWs is crucial. Debates persist regarding whether external funding for link worker salaries poses an obstacle to their development through training (Spencer et al., 2022).

All these factors highlighted, underscore the imperative for a nuanced comprehension of the financial structures, job evaluation, scope of practice supporting the role of SPLWs, how they intersect with training and professional growth, recruitment and retention and quality of service provision.

CHAPTER 4

Case Studies from Practice

This chapter will explore the real-life application of the Social Prescribing Link Worker model. Through three case studies, we will see the impact of Social Prescribing Link Workers (SPLWs) and where their influence may extend. It is noteworthy that the highlighted services garnered recognition through the competitive NALW award process, open to all participants across the UK within specified categories.

It is essential to clarify that the presented cases, while exemplary, are not exhaustive. As emphasised in the preface of this book, our intent is not to provide a comprehensive overview of all social prescribing models. Rather, these case studies serve as a focused exploration, offering nuanced insights into select services. The objective is to provide a detailed understanding of the operational dynamics of SPLW services, offering practical insights for diverse healthcare contexts.

■ Central Liverpool Primary Care Network (PCN)
Introduction

Central Liverpool Primary Care Network (CLPCN) is a member network of nine practices serving a patient footprint of 120,000 patients – the most ethnically diverse PCN in the heart of Liverpool. Around 23.5% of Central Liverpool's population are living in income deprived households and it is the fourth most deprived area nationally, with 36% of patients being Black or Asian and 17% having a language other than English as their first – the highest in Liverpool (Ministry of Housing, Communities and Local Government, 2019). CLPCN has a collective workforce of around 400 staff with a mission to reduce racial inequalities faced by patients and communities through accountability, population engagement and systematic collaboration. CLPCN's ambition is to create an inclusive, holistic healthcare journey for every patient.

In 2019 CLPCN began its journey towards recruiting for a robust social prescribing model and since then the PCN has gone on to employ seven SPLWs and 2.8 Work Time Equivalent (WTE) Network Engagement Leads.

Social Prescribing Intervention

The social prescribing model has a two-pronged approach, both encompassing direct employment of the SPLWs. The model allows for a referral pathway into the team whereby the SPLW works closely following a personalised care approach to supporting patients. Patients have multiple social, economic, and environmental issues that impact on their health. SPLWs have more time to focus on these factors with people, and on preventative work and empowerment. SPLWs promote equality, especially to people and groups where improvements in health and well-being are not in keeping with the rest of the population.

The second stream of social prescribing is done via the Network Engagement Leads approach, whose focus is mainly to thread the voice of our global majority patients into service delivery. The engagement leads have been instrumental in the production of key administrative tools to support access and improving patient satisfaction when accessing primary care services. The team have a clear working remit to integrate their skillsets in community asset development and support stakeholders, encouraging partnership and co-production work.

Impact

Year on year CLPCN have averaged around 1,400 referrals into the service alone, there is also a steady increase in patients being supported. In late 2022, a GP led social prescribing drop in session specifically for refugee and asylum seeker patient groups, was set up to meet local needs. SPLWs help ease workload and pressure on practices allowing clinicians to focus on the more clinical aspects of their work and provide referral routes for all practice staff.

They have been recognised locally and nationally for some of their innovative approaches to COVID-19 vaccination, including pop-up clinics in community venues and visits to asylum seeker, traveller and homeless populations. CLPCN use vaccination and other health events as opportunities to promote proactive SPLW services and take referrals, for example, the recent health event for International Women's Day at the PAL Centre on 8 March 2022. Their SPLWs also promote the new CLPCN community grant scheme to strengthen links with community partners and improve the range of services and support for their patients.

In 2022 the PCN reinvested £10,000 into local community groups/assets with encouraging feedback obtained. There are further plans for 2023/2024 to further reinvest £20,000. The PCN has received various qualitative narratives following on from this:

'CLPCN has really supported us here in being able to continue our vital work. We support people getting out into the local community and love where they live. Thank you.'

'Absolutely revolutionary. I can't tell you how amazing you and your team have been. In situations where it felt like there was nothing to do or offer to patients you have been a beacon of hope! Amazing.' – Doctor

'The social prescribing and well-being team have been a vital source of help for our patients, especially as mental health has worsened due to the pandemic. I have been informed by multiple patients they have valued their help.'– Doctor

'I have been thrilled with this service and it has massively exceeded my very highest expectations. You and your team have done a great job in supporting our patients with often very complex physical emotional and social problems compounded by living in poverty and have been great enablers. I'm not sure how we managed without you!' – Doctor

'I remember that one patient told me that you had changed her life with your help and support about one and a half years ago.' – Doctor

'I think the service you offer is absolutely fantastic. There is such a need for this especially in deprived areas where people experience such enormous social stressors which affect their health.'

'I think patients often feel completely overwhelmed by their issues. When they come to the GP we have to try and manage their medical and mental health problems, but we know that if they are in debt, have issues with their housing or are lonely for example, their physical health takes a back seat and they are unlikely to improve. Being able to refer to yourself adds so much to patient care and I think improves their outcomes massively.' – Doctor

In 2022 CLPCN went on to win the National Association Link Workers', Social Prescribing Employer of the Year Award.

■ North East London Health & Care Partnership

Setting

NHS North East London (NEL), also known as the North East London Health and Care Partnership (NEL HCP), is the integrated care board for a population of almost two million, including some of the most disadvantaged communities in the UK. The pandemic and soaring cost of living have profoundly impacted health in the area, exacerbating health inequalities and service pressures.

Social Prescribing Intervention

NEL has established a powerful social prescribing partnership over the last three years, founded on extensive engagement with frontline teams at the outset of the pandemic. The programme was founded on inclusive and caring leadership principles, supporting their link workers to realise their potential in order to unlock the power of our communities.

Their model was co-designed with link workers and co-produced with local community groups, key leaders from across their place-based partnerships (PBPs), including statutory and voluntary sector partners. The enthusiastic buy-in meant there are now 95+ social prescribing link workers in primary care networks (PCNs), boroughs and the voluntary sector in North East London. They have established a foundation for social prescribing through evaluation, workforce development and community chests, that has transformed care in North East London, with learning shared extensively with regional and national teams.

Impact

Uptake of social prescribing across the partnership has almost trebled over the last two years (from 15,418 unique patient referrals in 2020 to 42,635 in 2022) and user feedback shows it is making an immense difference to the lives of their residents.

Working with link workers, managers, GPs, PBPs and PCNs, they developed a personalised care minimum dataset with an easy-to-use social prescribing dashboard. All teams can see at a glance the demographics of those accessing social prescribing and get an idea of why. This work helped to shape the national minimum dataset, developed by NHS England.

With logistical and facilitative support from the partnership, all boroughs and place-based partnerships are running Community Chests for social prescribing totalling more than £400,000. These are equity-centred micro-funds for local groups, enabling them to deliver activities and services that meet the needs of underserved communities, street by street and neighbourhood by neighbourhood.

They are the first London integrated care board to take a system-wide, co-produced, partnered approach to funding and delivering activities linked to social prescribing, and are sharing learning via an eleven-part toolkit. In 2022, they won the National Association of Link Workers Social Prescribing Workforce initiative of the year award recognising their emerging leaders programme for link workers.

■ Health and Social Care Alliance Scotland (ALLIANCE)

Setting

The ALLIANCE Links Worker Programme is an established social prescribing force delivering across two Scottish local authority areas, offering targeted support to participants and assisting GPs across nearly 70 practices. The ALLIANCE has been employing link workers since early 2014 when the programme started in seven Deep End GP practices across Glasgow.

Initially funded by Scottish Government as a two-year pilot programme it is now funded by Glasgow City Health and Social Care Partnership (HSCP). They secured the contract with West Dunbartonshire in the summer of 2021 where funding is initially for three years through Primary Care Improvement Plan monies governed by the HSCP and local authority.

Social Prescribing Intervention

A Community Link Worker (CLW) is a community orientated role, in this case attached to one or more Primary Care Teams (PCTs), whose principal purpose is to assist people to access community resources that will support them to live well.

Within Glasgow the model is made up of two inter-related interventions: the provision of a link worker, attached to a practice and the development of a Links Approach by the practice team. The interventions target GP practices in areas of high socio-economic deprivation. Working in a person-centred manner, the CLW will work with anyone registered with the GP practice in which they are hosted, they will arrange appointments in a setting suitable to the individual and have hour-long appointments. There is no time limit on how long someone can work with the CLW, as working with a person-centred approach ensures that the issues the individual wishes to address are discussed. The average number of appointments is four, but this can vary from one to over 20 appointments. The three main issues that individuals wish to address are mental health, income related issues, housing and poverty. Many other issues are also highlighted such as bereavement, relationship issues and loneliness.

In West Dunbartonshire the model is very similar in the approach and provision of a CLW, the only difference is appointments are 30 minutes (although double appointments can be arranged if required).

Across both programmes the ALLIANCE employ 66 staff within the Links Worker Programme.

Impact

Over 9,000 people across Glasgow and West Dunbartonshire engaged with a Community Link Worker (CLW) in 2022 and in the same time frame over 35,000 appointments took place. This included over 6,800 in-person appointments, as part of a gradual transition to a 'new normal', though it is expected that going forward telephone interactions will be a greater part of a CLW's diary than it was before the pandemic. CLWs continue to deal with a wide range of issues, with the cost-of-living crisis becoming a particular focus towards the end of the year.

The Social Prescribing Link Worker Model

CLWs link in with a variety of community and statutory organisations as part of the link process and work closely to ensure referral pathways and access to services meet the needs of those they are working alongside.

> 'Thank you for helping me through the whole situation with the house thing. Now I am able to live with my partner, today my housing came and told me that now I can live with my partner and his kids, thank you so much once again.' – Participant

> 'All I can say is that [CLW] is a breath of fresh air. Having someone with [their] energy and [their] young attitude is what we need.' – Practice Manager

> 'Thank you for your work, feedback from patients has been great.' – GP

> 'Any worries I have I know I can ask you and you'll point me in the right direction.' –Participant

In 2022, one of our Community Link Workers won, the National Association of Link Workers', Link Worker of the Year award.

Steadfast in our commitment to a healthcare paradigm that is not only curative but, more importantly, preventive, holistic, person and community-centred on the well-being of individuals and societies. Social prescribing stands as a beacon, guiding us towards a future where health is a state of flourishing for all.

> 'Social prescribing is probably the 'biggest cultural shift' in medicine and healthcare for generations, but more needs to be done to realise its benefits'.
>
> Prof Martin Marshall, Chair of Royal College of General Practitioners, 2021) (quoted in GP Online, 2021).

Conclusion and Reflections

■ Conclusion

As we conclude this book, it becomes apparent that we are standing at the precipice of a transformative era in healthcare. The journey we have undertaken has revealed the intricate dynamics, challenges and potential of the Social Prescribing Link Worker model.

The role of Social Prescribing Link Workers (SPLWs) has evolved and continues to evolve, requiring ongoing support and sustainability. To propel this practice into the future, the next steps must be intentional and collaborative. Addressing the National Association of Link Workers' (NALW) research priorities is essential, along with delivering on the Royal College of General Practitioners' (RCGP) 2018 call for a social prescriber in every practice. Ensuring adequate training, supervision and defining the scope of practice are critical aspects.

Policymakers play a pivotal role in fully integrating social prescribing into the fabric of healthcare systems. Developing guidelines for seamless integration into existing healthcare structures and policies that support the long-term sustainability of social prescribing is paramount. Support with funding, regulation and training of workers is crucial to facilitate integration into other parts of the primary care ecosystem, such as pharmacy, ensuring a no-wrong-door approach within the healthcare system and cross-sectoral working.

Embracing this cultural change requires a commitment to adaptability, innovation, and a collective stance for the common good of society. As we move forward, general practitioners, SPLWs, health and care practitioners, policymakers, academics, researchers, and the broader community will need to continue to demand and drive the cultural shift. Progress should include evolving the training curriculum for medical, health and care professions to include a social prescribing model. Whilst this is already happening in some institutions, it is not universal. In order to embed this into the training for those already qualified, CPD opportunities should also include social prescribing, and this something professional bodies and statutory bodes can help drive.

Conclusion and Reflections

The challenges encountered on this journey are not roadblocks but rather opportunities for growth. Conflicts of interest, short-term focuses, power struggles, culture wars, and protectionist tendencies can be addressed through a collective commitment to sustained behavioural changes, transparency and a shared vision of healthcare as a dynamic and adaptive ecosystem.

The role of technology in the future of social prescribing cannot be understated. Leveraging digital tools, therapeutics and data analytics can enhance the efficiency, reach and impact of social prescribing, population health management and data-driven commissioning, funding the entire patient journey remains critical for success.

In a world characterised by social and economic inequalities, public health emergencies, conflicts, and the looming climate crisis, the importance of social prescribing link workers is poised to grow significantly. Global structural threats to mental health, as highlighted by the World Health Organisation (WHO, 2022b), underscore the critical need for interventions that help address multifaceted challenges, recognising that well-being extends beyond medical interventions.

Looking ahead, the role of social prescribing link workers will continue to evolve in tandem with the shifting dynamics of our world. As societies grapple with complex issues, social prescribing link workers emerge as indispensable figures whose potential needs to be maximised and supported, and whose role deserves recognition, full support, and regulation to prevent social prescribing from being jeopardised. The future of social prescribing hinges on a collective effort, necessitating active participation from health and care professionals, researchers, policymakers, patients, and communities alike. This collaborative approach is vital to effectively address the challenges presented by a complex and ever-evolving world.

Reflections

We have covered a lot in this book, from the challenges that face healthcare and the context of the SPLW service, workforce, benefits, challenges, and benchmark tools to practical applications. What are your key takeaways from this book? We would love to hear your thoughts.

Bibliography

Adams-Prassl A et al. (2022) The impact of the coronavirus lockdown on mental health: evidence from the United States. *Economic Policy*, 37(109): 139–155.

Adler K (2018) Screening for Social Determinants of Health: An Opportunity or Unreasonable Burden? *Family Practice Management*, 25(3): 3

Barnett K et al. (2012) Epidemiology of multimorbidity and implications for health care, research, and medical education: a cross-sectional study. *The Lancet*, 380(9836): 37–43.

Bhatti S et al. (2021) Using self-determination theory to understand the social prescribing process: a qualitative study. *BJGP Open*, 5(2): BJGPO.2020.0153.

Bickerdike L et al. (2017) Social prescribing: less rhetoric and more reality. A systematic review of the evidence. *BMJ Open*, 7(4): e013384.

Blockley K et al. (2020) What approaches to social prescribing work, for whom, and in what circumstances? A realist review. *Health and Social Care in the Community*, 28(2): 309–324.

BMA (2023a) Save our surgeries. Available at: https://www.bma.org.uk/advice-and-support/nhs-delivery-and-workforce/pressures/wales-save-our-surgeries-campaign [accessed 28 November 2023].

BMA (2023b) 80% of GPs express patient safety concerns as GP crisis deepens in Wales. Available at: https://www.bma.org.uk/bma-media-centre/80-of-gps-express-patient-safety-concerns-as-gp-crisis-deepens-in-wales [accessed 28 November 2023].

BMA (2023c) The sustainability crisis in GP practice in Scotland. Available at: https://www.bma.org.uk/advice-and-support/gp-practices/funding-and-contracts/the-sustainability-crisis-in-gp-practice-in-scotland [accessed 28 November 2023].

BMA (2023d) Safe working in general practice. Available at: https://www.bma.org.uk/advice-and-support/gp-practices/managing-workload/safe-working-in-general-practice [accessed 28 November 2023].

Bibliography

BMA (2023e) Safe working for GPs in Northern Ireland. Available at: https://www.bma.org.uk/advice-and-support/gp-practices/managing-workload/safe-working-for-gps-in-northern-ireland [accessed 28 November 2023].

BMA (2023f) Annual Conference of England LMC Representatives. Available at: https://www.bma.org.uk/media/7762/agenda-england-lmc-conference-final-nov-2023.pdf [accessed 28 March 2024].

BMA (2021) NHS medical staffing data analysis. Available at: https://www.bma.org.uk/advice-and-support/nhs-delivery-and-workforce/workforce/nhs-medical-staffing-data-analysis [accessed 29 March 2023].

British Red Cross (2021) Nowhere else to turn. Available at: https://www.redcross.org.uk/about-us/what-we-do/we-speak-up-for-change/exploring-the-high-intensity-use-of-accident-and-emergency-services [accessed 18 November 2022].

Cacioppo J T and Cacioppo S (2014) Older adults reporting social isolation or loneliness show poorer cognitive function 4 years later. *Evidence-based nursing*, 17(2): 59–60.

Calderón-Larrañaga S, Greenhalgh T and Clinch M (2023) Unravelling the potential of social prescribing in individual-level type 2 diabetes prevention: a mixed-methods realist evaluation. *BMC Med* (21)91. Available at: https://doi.org/10.1186/s12916-023-02796-9.

Centre for Mental Health (2021) Better together. Available at: https://www.centreformentalhealth.org.uk/publications/briefing-57-better-together [accessed 18 November 2022].

Chang J E et al. (2021) Rapid transition to telehealth and the digital divide: Implications for primary care access and equity in a post-COVID era. *The Milbank Quarterly*, 99(2): 340–368.

Cohen J and Ezer T (2013) Human rights in patient care: a theoretical and practical framework. *Health and Human Rights*, (15)2: 7–19.

Cooper M et al. (2022) Effectiveness and active ingredients of social prescribing interventions targeting mental health: a systematic review, *BMJ Open*, 12: e060214. Available at: doi: 10.1136/bmjopen-2021-060214.

Costa A et al. (2021) Developing a social prescribing local system in a European Mediterranean country: a feasibility study to promote active and healthy aging. *BMC Health Services Research*, 21(1): 1164.

Cruwys T et al. (2018) Social isolation predicts frequent attendance in primary care. *Annals of Behavioral Medicine*, 52(10): 817–829.

Department of Health and Social Care (2021) Good for you, good for us, good for everybody. Available at: https://assets.publishing.service.gov.uk/government/uploads/system/uploads/attachment_data/file/1019475/good-for-you-good-for-us-good-for-everybody.pdf [accessed 13 December 2022].

Department of Health and Social Care (2019) Social prescribing: new national academy set up. Available at: https://www.gov.uk/government/news/social-prescribing-new-national-academy-set-up [accessed 18 November 2022].

Bibliography

Doblytė S (2020) Under- or overtreatment of mental distress? Practices, consequences, and resistance in the field of mental health care. *Qualitative Health Research*, 30(10): 1503–1516. Available at: doi:10.1177/1049732320918531 [accessed 5 January 2024]

Eden Project (2017) The cost of disconnected communities. Available at: https://www.edenprojectcommunities.com/blog/the-cost-of-disconnected-communities#:~:text=A%20study%20has%20found%20that%20disconnected%20communities%20could,services%20of%20social%20isolation%20and%20disconnected%20communities%2C%20including%3A [accessed 25 November 2022].

Elston J et al. (2019) Does a social prescribing 'holistic' link-worker for older people with complex, multimorbidity improve well-being and frailty and reduce health and social care use and costs? A 12-month before-and-after evaluation. *Primary Health Care Research & Development*, 20: e135.

Engel G L (1977) The need for a new medical model: a challenge for biomedicine. *Science*, 196(4286): 129–136. Available at: https://www.ncbi.nlm.nih.gov/pmc/articles/PMC4062058/ [accessed 5 January 2024].

Evers S et al (2024) Theories used to develop or evaluate social prescribing in studies: a scoping review. *BMC Health Serv Res*, 24(1):140. Available at: https://pubmed.ncbi.nlm.nih.gov/38279096/ [accessed 28 March 2024].

Fixsen A and Barrett S (2022) Challenges and approaches to green social prescribing suring and in the aftermath of COVID-19: A qualitative study. *Frontiers In Psychology*, 13: 861107.

Foster A et al. (2021) Impact of social prescribing to address loneliness: A mixed methods evaluation of a national social prescribing programme. *Health and Social Care Community*; 29: 1439–1449. Available at: https://doi.org/10.1111/hsc.13200.

Frostick C and Bertotti M (2021) The frontline of social prescribing – How do we ensure link workers can work safely and effectively within primary care? *Chronic Illness*; 17(4): 404–415. Available at: https://doi.org/10.1177/1742395319882068 [accessed 5 January 2024].

Galway K et al. (2019) Adapting digital social prescribing for suicide bereavement support: the findings of a consultation exercise to explore the acceptability of implementing digital social prescribing within an existing postvention service. *International Journal of Environmental Research and Public Health*, 16(22): 4561.

Garzón-Orjuela et al. (2020) An overview of reviews on strategies to reduce health inequalities. *International Journal for Equity in Health*, 19(1).

Gilbert-Johns S et al. (2022) Overview of the UK population: 2020. *Office for National Statistics*. Available at: https://www.ons.gov.uk/peoplepopulationandcommunity/populationandmigration/populationestimates/articles/overviewoftheukpopulation/2020 [accessed 18 November 2022].

Bibliography

GP Online (2021) Social prescribing is 'biggest cultural shift' in medicine for generations, says RCGP chair. Available at: https://www.gponline.com/social-prescribing-biggest-cultural-shift-medicine-generations-says-rcgp-chair/article/1729825 [accessed 5 January 2024].

Hassan SM et al. (2020) Social prescribing for people with mental health needs living in disadvantaged communities: The Life Rooms model. *BMC Health Serv Res*, (20)19.

Husk K et al. (2019) Social prescribing: where is the evidence? *The British Journal of General Practice*, 69(678): 6–7. Available at: https://bjgp.org/content/69/678/6. [accessed 5 January 2024].

International Conference on Primary Health Care (1978) Declaration of Alma-Ata. *WHO Chronicle*, 32(11): 428–430.

Johnston M C et al. (2019) Defining and measuring multimorbidity: a systematic review of systematic reviews, *European Journal of Public Health*, 29(1): 182–189. Available at: https://doi.org/10.1093/eurpub/cky098 [accessed 5 January 2024].

Kiely B et al. (2022) Effect of social prescribing link workers on health outcomes and costs for adults in primary care and community settings: a systematic review. *BMJ Open*, 12(10): e062951.

Kiely B et al. (2021) Link workers providing social prescribing and health and social care coordination for people with multimorbidity in socially deprived areas (the LinkMM trial): protocol for a pragmatic randomised controlled trial. *BMJ Open*, 11(2): e041809.

Leigh-Hunt N et al. (2017) An overview of systematic reviews on the public health consequences of social isolation and loneliness. *Public Health*, 152: 157–171.

Marmot, M, Goldblatt P, Allen J et al. (2010) Fair Society, Healthy Lives (The Marmot report). Institute of Health Equity. Available at: https://www.instituteofhealthequity.org/resources-reports/fair-society-healthy-lives-the-marmot-review [accessed 5 January 2024].

Marmot M and Allen J (2020) COVID-19: exposing and amplifying inequalities. *Journal of Epidemiology and Community Health*, 74(9): 681–682. Available at: https://jech.bmj.com/content/74/9/681 [accessed 5 January 2024].

McClellan, H et al. (2020) Loneliness as a predictor of suicidal ideation and behaviour: a systematic review and meta-analysis of prospective studies. *Journal of Affective Disorders* (274): 880–896. Available at: https://pubmed.ncbi.nlm.nih.gov/32669357/ [accessed 5 January 2024].

Mercer SW et al. (2019). The GP as a prescriber. *British Journal of General Practice*, 69(679): 6–7.

Ministry of Housing, Communities and Local Government (2019) The English Indices of Deprivation 2019 (IoD2019). Available at: https://assets.publishing.service.gov.uk/media/5d8e26f6ed915d5570c6cc55/IoD2019_Statistical_Release.pdf [accessed 5 January 2024].

Bibliography

Moffatt, S et al. (2017) Link worker social prescribing to improve health and well-being for people with long-term conditions: qualitative study of service user perceptions. *BMJ Open*, 7(7): e015203.

Moore C et al. (2023) 'Winging it': An exploration of the self-perceived professional identity of social prescribing link workers. *Health & Social Care in the Community*. Available at: https://doi.org/10.1155/2023/8488615 [accessed 5 January 2024].

National Association of Link Workers (NALW) (2023a) Exploring social prescribing referrals and impact on information, advice and guidance services. Available at.https://www.nalw.org.uk/wp-content/uploads/2023/05/Exploring-Social-Prescribing-Referrals-_-impact-on-Information_-Advice-and-Guidance-Services_Research-Report.pdf [accessed 29 March 2023].

National Association of Link Workers (NALW) (2023b) Supervision guidance for social prescribing link workers and supervisors. Available at: https://www.nalw.org.uk/supervision/ [accessed 5 January 2024].

National Association of Link Workers (NALW) (2022a) Code of practice for employers of social prescribing link workers and social prescribing link workers. Available at: https://www.nalw.org.uk/wp-content/uploads/2022/05/NALW_Code-of-Practice-for-employers-of-social-prescribing-link-workers-and-social-prescribing-link-workers_May-2022.pdf [accessed 4 December 2022].

National Association of Link Workers (NALW) (2022b) Education standards for social prescribing link workers. Available at: https://www.nalw.org.uk/wp-content/uploads/2022/05/NALW-Education-Standards-For-Social-Prescribing-Link-Workers_May-2022.pdf [accessed 4 December 2022].

National Association of Link Workers (NALW) (2022c) Implementation of the social prescribing link worker role in elective care. Available at: https://www.nalw.org.uk/wp-content/uploads/2022/11/NALW-Case-Study-Elective-care.pdf [accessed 27 December 2022].

National Association of Link Workers (NALW) (2022d) Workplace supervision with a GP. Available at: https://www.nalw.org.uk/supervision-resources/ [accessed 29 March 2023].

National Association of Link Workers (NALW) (2022e) World Mental Health Day: Making Mental health and wellbeing (Social Prescribing) for ALL a global priority. Available at: https://www.nalw.org.uk/world-mental-health-day-making-mental-health-social-prescribing-for-all-a-global-priority/ [accessed 20 November 2022].

National Association of Link Workers (NALW (2022f) The role of Patient Participation Groups (PPGs) in social prescribing: PPGs perspective on awareness and collaboration with Link Workers. Available at https://www.nalw.org.uk/wp-content/uploads/2022/05/The-Role-of-PPGs-in-Social-Prescribing.pdf"The-Role-of-PPGs-in-Social-Prescribing.pdf [accessed 4 February 2024].

Bibliography

National Association of Link Workers (NALW) (2022g) Supervision types for social prescribing link workers: social prescribing supervision short films. Available at: https://www.nalw.org.uk/supervision-resources/ [accessed 29 March 2023].

National Association of Link Workers (NALW) (2021a). NALW Response to the Personalised Care Group at NHSE/I's request for consultation on the professional Registration of Health and Wellbeing Coaches, Care Coordinators and Social Prescribing Link Workers (March/April 2021). Available at: https://www.nalw.org.uk/wp-content/uploads/2021/04/NALW-Professional-Register-Consultation-Response-Survey-Report-20th-April-2021.pdf [accessed 25 November 2022].

National Association of Link Workers (NALW) (2021b). NHS Confed Conference briefing: mental health in the time of COVID-19: The system response. Available at: https://www.nalw.org.uk/development/nhs-confed-conference-mental-health-in-the-time-of-covid-19-the-system-response/ [accessed 20 November 2022].

National Association of Link Workers (NALW) (2021c) The role of social prescribing link workers in reducing health inequalities. Available at: https://www.nalw.org.uk/wp-content/uploads/2021/10/Role-of-Social-Prescribing-Link-Workers-in-reducing-Health-Inequalities-8th-October-2021.pdf [accessed 18 November 2022].

National Association of Link Workers (NALW) (2020a) Book of social prescribing link workers impact. Available at: https://www.nalw.org.uk/wp-content/uploads/2020/10/Released-LinkWorkerDay2020-Book-of-Social-Prescribing-Link-Workers-Impact.pdf [accessed 22 December 2022].

National Association of Link Workers (NALW) (2020b) Care for the carer: Social prescribing link workers views, perspectives, and experiences of clinical supervision and wellbeing support. Available at: https://www.nalw.org.uk/wp-content/uploads/2020/07/NALW_Care-for-the-Carer_-Report_8th-July-2020-Final.pdf [accessed 4 December 2022].

National Association of Link Workers (NALW) (2019a) Getting to know the link worker workforce: Understanding link workers knowledge, skills, experiences, and support needs. Available at: https://www.nalw.org.uk/wp-content/uploads/2019/06/Released_NALW_link-worker-report_March-2019_updated.pdf [accessed 4 December 2022].

National Association of Link Workers (NALW) (2019b) Peer group clinical supervision: review and evaluation. Available at: https://nalw.org.uk/wp-content/uploads/2019/12/Released_NALW_Peer-Group-Clinical-Supervision_Review-and-Evaluation.pdf [accessed 4 December 2022].

NHS (2023) Workforce development framework: social prescribing link workers. Available at: https://www.england.nhs.uk/long-read/workforce-development-framework-social-prescribing-link-workers/ [accessed 29 March 2023].

NHS (2019) The NHS long term plan. Available at: https://www.longtermplan.nhs.uk/publication/nhs-long-term-plan/ [accessed 18 November 2022].

Bibliography

NHS Business Services Authority (NHSBSA) (2022) Medicines used in mental health – England: 2015/16 to 2021/22. Available at: https://www.nhsbsa.nhs.uk/statistical-collections/medicines-used-mental-health-england/medicines-used-mental-health-england-201516-202122 [accessed 19 November 2022].

NHS Confederation (2020) How health and care systems can work better with VCSE partners. Available at: https://www.nhsconfed.org/publications/how-health-and-care-systems-can-work-better-vcse-partners [accessed 25 November 2022].

NHS Digital (2018) Statistics on obesity, physical activity and diet: England, 2018 [PAS]. Available at: https://digital.nhs.uk/data-and-information/publications/statistical/statistics-on-obesity-physical-activity-and-diet/statistics-on-obesity-physical-activity-and-diet-england-2018 [accessed 18 November 2022].

NHS England (2023) Primary Care Network workforce, 28 February 2023. Available at: https://digital.nhs.uk/data-and-information/publications/statistical/primary-care-network-workforce/28-february-2023 [accessed 29 March 2023].

NHS England (2024) NHS long-term plan workforce plan. Available at: https://www.england.nhs.uk/long-read/nhs-long-term-workforce-plan-2/#4-reform-working-and-training-differently [accessed 29 March 2023].

NHS England (2022a) Green social prescribing. Available at: https://www.england.nhs.uk/personalisedcare/social-prescribing/green-social-prescribing/ [accessed 20 November 2022].

NHS England (2022b) Voluntary, community and social enterprises (VCSE). Available at: https://www.england.nhs.uk/ourwork/part-rel/voluntary-community-and-social-enterprises-vcse/ [accessed 25 November 2022].

NHS England (2022c) Working in partnership with people and communities. Statutory guidance. Available at: https://www.england.nhs.uk/wp-content/uploads/2022/07/B1762-guidance-on-working-in-partnership-with-people-and-communities.pdf [accessed 25 November 2022].

NHS England (2021) Social prescribing link worker. Available at: https://www.healthcareers.nhs.uk/explore-roles/wider-healthcare-team/roles-wider-healthcare-team/clinical-support-staff/social-prescribing-link-worker/social-prescribing-link-worker [accessed 25 November 2022].

NHS England (2017a) 1.4 million people referred to NHS mental health therapy in the past year. Available at: https://www.england.nhs.uk/2017/12/1-4-million-people-referred-to-nhs-mental-health-therapy-in-the-past-year/ [accessed 18 November 2022].

NHS England (2017b) Next steps on the NHS Five Year Forward View. Available at: https://www.england.nhs.uk/publication/next-steps-on-the-nhs-five-year-forward-view/ [accessed 18 November 2022].

Nuffield Trust (2022) The long goodbye? Exploring rates of staff leaving the NHS and social care. Available at: https://www.nuffieldtrust.org.uk/resource/the-long-goodbye-exploring-rates-of-staff-leaving-the-nhs-and-social-care [accessed 20 November 2022].

Bibliography

Office for National Statistics (2021a) Mapping loneliness during the coronavirus pandemic. Available at: https://www.ons.gov.uk/peoplepopulationandcommunity/wellbeing/articles/mappinglonelinessduringthecoronaviruspandemic/2021-04-07 [accessed 20 November 2022].

Office for National Statistics (2021b) *Suicides in England and Wales: 2021 registrations*. Available at: https://www.ons.gov.uk/peoplepopulationandcommunity/birthsdeathsandmarriages/deaths/bulletins/suicidesintheunitedkingdom/2021registrations [accessed 20 November 2022].

Tammes P et al. (2021) Is continuity of primary care declining in England? Practice-level longitudinal study from 2012 to 2017. *British Journal of General Practice 2021*, 71(707): e432-e440. Available at: doi: 10.3399/BJGP.2020.0935

The Pioneer Health Foundation (2022) The Peckham Experiment. Available at: https://thephf.org/peckhamexperiment [accessed 18 November 2022].

Polley M J et al. (2020) What does successful social prescribing look like? Mapping meaningful outcomes. Available at: https://westminsterresearch.westminster.ac.uk/item/qyz67/what-does-successful-social-prescribing-look-like-mapping-meaningful-outcomes [accessed 29 March 2023].

Polley M et al. [On behalf of the NASP Academic Partners Collaborative] (2022) Measuring outcomes for individuals receiving support through social prescribing. *National Academy for Social Prescribing*. Available at: https://socialprescribingacademy.org.uk/media/kp3lhrhv/evidence-review-measuring-impact-and-outcomes-for-social-prescribing.pdf [accessed 5 January 2024].

Punton G, Dodd A L and McNeill A (2022) 'You're on the waiting list': An interpretive phenomenological analysis of young adults' experiences of waiting lists within mental health services in the UK. *PLOS ONE*, 17(3): e0265542. Available at: https://doi.org/10.1371/journal.pone.0265542.

Professional Records Standards Body (PRSB) 2022. *Social Prescribing Information Standard*. Available at: https://theprsb.org/standards/social-prescribing-standard/ [accessed 08 December 2022].

Public Health Scotland (2021) What are health inequalities? Available at: https://www.healthscotland.scot/health-inequalities/what-are-health-inequalities [accessed 18 November 2022].

Reinhardt G Y, Vidovic D and Hammerton C (2021) Understanding loneliness: a systematic review of the impact of social prescribing initiatives on loneliness. *Perspectives in Public Health*, 141(4): 204–213.

Rhodes, J and Bell, S (2021) 'It sounded a lot simpler on the job description': A qualitative study exploring the role of social prescribing link workers and their training and support needs. *Health and Social Care Community*, 29: e338–e347. Available at: https://doi.org/10.1111/hsc.13358.

Bibliography

Royal College of General Practitioners (2018) Loneliness: Manifesto. Available at: https://www.rcgp.org.uk/representing-you/policy-areas/loneliness [accessed 8 March 2024].

Royal College of Psychiatrists (2021) Combat the mental health fallout of COVID-19 by improving access to social prescribing, say Royal Colleges. Available at: https://www.rcpsych.ac.uk/news-and-features/latest-news/detail/2021/03/18/combat-the-mental-health-fallout-of-covid-19-by-improving-access-to-social-prescribing-say-royal-colleges [accessed 20 November 2022].

Sandhu S et al. (2022). Intervention components of link worker social prescribing programmes: A scoping review. *Health and Social Care in the Community*, 30: e3761–e3774. Available at: https://doi.org/10.1111/hsc.14056 [accessed 5 January 2024].

Scottish Government (2022) Increasing mental health support in GP practices. Available at: https://www.gov.scot/news/increasing-mental-health-support-in-gp-practices/ [accessed 20 November 2022].

Scottish Parliament. Health, Social Care and Sport Committee (2022) Alternative pathways to primary care. Available at: https://digitalpublications.parliament.scot/Committees/Report/HSCS/2022/6/17/0e05bfbf-b984-4031-97ee-6129de863e93#dba79965-3dc5-4658-b2e3-4a17d671f000.dita [accessed 29 March 2023].

Scottish Government (2023) Primary care improvement plans: summary of implementation progress at March 2023. Available at: https://www.gov.scot/publications/primary-care-improvement-plans-summary-implementation-progress-march-2023/ [accessed 29 January 2024].

Skivington K et al. (2021) A new framework for developing and evaluating complex interventions: update of Medical Research Council guidance. *BMJ*: n2061.

Spencer L H et al. (2022) Qualifications and training needs of social prescribing link workers: an explorative study. *The Lancet*, 400(S79). Available at: https://doi.org/10.1016/S0140-6736(22)02289-9 [accessed 5 January 2024].

SPRING (2023) SPRING social prescribing project Available at: https://www.tnlcommunityfund.org.uk/media/insights/documents/SPRING-2023-Evaluation-Final-1023.pdf?mtime=20240111100551&focal=none [accessed 5 January 2024].

Tierney S et al. (2022) Social prescribing for older people and the role of the cultural sector during the COVID-19 pandemic: What are link workers' views and experiences? *Health and Social Care in the Community*. Available at: https://doi.org/10.1111/hsc.13949 [accessed 5 January 2024].

Tierney S et al. (2020) Supporting social prescribing in primary care by linking people to local assets: a realist review. *BMC Medicine*, 18(49). Available at: https://doi.org/10.1186/s12916-020-1510-7 [accessed 5 January 2024].

UK Research and Innovation (no date). COVID-19 and VCSE organisations response. Available at: https://gtr.ukri.org/projects?ref=ES%2FV007610%2F1 [accessed 25 November 2022].

Bibliography

UNISON (2023) Health Care Service Group Conference. Available at: https://www.unison.org.uk/events/2023-health-care-sg-conference/ [accessed 28 March 2024]. https://www.unison.org.uk/content/uploads/2023/03/2023-Health-Conference-Final-Agenda-and-Guide.pdf link to the motion

University of Oxford (2022) Fostering connections between social prescribing link workers and the cultural sector. Available at: https://www.ox.ac.uk/research/research-impact/fostering-connections-between-social-prescribing-link-workers-and-cultural [accessed 13 December 2022].

Wallace E et al. (2015) Managing patients with multimorbidity in primary care. *BMJ*, 350: h176. Available at: doi: 10.1136/bmj.h176. PMID: 25646760. [accessed 5 January 2024].

Wallace C et al. (2021). Understanding social prescribing in Wales: A mixed methods study. *Wales School for Social Prescribing Research (WSSPR)*. Available at: http://www.wsspr.wales/resources/PHW_SP_Report_FINAL.pdf [accessed 5 January 2024].

Watt T et al. (2023) Health in 2040: Projected patterns of illness in England. The Health Foundation; 2023. Available at: https://www.health.org.uk/publications/health-in-2040 [accessed 5 January 2024].

Welsh Government (2022) Consultation launched to provide good access to social prescribing across Wales. Available at: https://gov.wales/consultation-launched-provide-good-access-social-prescribing-across-wales [accessed 20 November 2022].

Welsh Government (2023). National framework for social prescribing. Available at: https://www.gov.wales/national-framework-social-prescribing [accessed 20 November 2022].

Woodall J et al. (2018) Understanding the effectiveness and mechanisms of a social prescribing service: a mixed method analysis. *BMC Health Services Research*, 18(1).

World Health Organization (2018). A vision for primary health care in the 21st century. Available: https://www.who.int/docs/default-source/primary-health/vision.pdf [accessed 5 January 2024].

World Health Organization (2022a). A toolkit on how to implement social prescribing. https://iris.who.int/bitstream/handle/10665/354456/9789290619765-eng.pdf?sequence=1 [accessed 5 January 2024].

World Health Organization (2022b). WHO highlights urgent need to transform mental health and mental health care. Available at: https://www.who.int/news/item/17-06-2022-who-highlights-urgent-need-to-transform-mental-health-and-mental-health-care [accessed 5 January 2024].

World Health Organization and United Nations Children's Fund (UNICEF) (2018) A vision for primary health care in the 21st century: towards universal health coverage and the sustainable development goals. Available at: https://apps.who.int/iris/handle/10665/328065 [accessed 18 November 2022].

Index

A
Alma-Ata Declaration of 1978, 7

B
Biopsychosocial model (BPS), 9
British Medical Association (BMA), 6

C
Central Liverpool Primary Care Network (PCN), 35–37
Chronic conditions, rise of, 2–3
COVID-19 pandemic, 4

D
Detriments of loneliness, 4

E
England, workforce challenges in, 6

H
Health and Social Care Alliance Scotland (ALLIANCE), 38–40
Healthcare challenges, 2–6
Health inequalities, 4–6

M
Mental health issues, 3–4
Multidisciplinary Teams (MDT), 10
Multimorbidity, 2

N
National Association of Link Workers (NALW), 22, 25
National Framework for Social Prescribing (NFfSP), 10
National Health Service (NHS), 9
North East London Health & Care Partnership, 37–38
Northern Ireland, workforce challenges in, 6

P
Primary Care Improvement Plan (PCIP), 10
Primary healthcare (PHC), 7–9
    components of, 8
Professional Record Standards Body (PRSB), 33
Professional supervision, 32

S
Scotland, workforce challenges in, 6
Social Prescribing Link Worker Model (SPLW), 11–24
    benefits and challenges in, 22–23
    biopsychosocial model, 9
    career path, 27
    case studies, 35–40

Index

Social Prescribing Link (*Continued*)
- codes of practice, 29–31
- as complex intervention, 23–24
- conclusion, 41–42
- COVID-19 pandemic, 4
- education standards, 31–32
- healthcare challenges, 2–6
- historical context, 7
- information standard, 33
- life of, 14–20
- overview, 11–12
- policy influences, 9–10
- primary care context, 7–9
- recruitment and retention, 33–34
- role, 21
- supervision, 32–33
- types, 28
- work, 12–13
- workforce challenges in general practice, 6
- workforce composition, 25–28

SPRING Social Prescribing Project, 10

V

Voluntary, community, and social enterprise (VCSE), 12, 21–22

W

Wales, workforce challenges in, 6

Workplace supervision, 32

World Health Organization (WHO)
- vision for 21st century primary care, 8–9